Tai Chi Sword

The 32 Simplified Forms

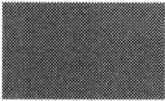

Other Books in the Tai Chi Series

Tai Chi for Health: The 24 Simplified Forms
    by Cheng Zhao & Don Zhao
    (ISBN 0-976118-31-9)

Tai Chi Sword

The 32 Simplified Forms

Li Guangqi
Cheng Zhao

Agilceed Books
Indiana, U.S.A.

Library of Congress Control Number (LCCN): 2006934441

TITILE Tai Chi Sword: The 32 Simplified Forms

ISBN-10: 0-9761183-2-7
ISBN-13: 978-0-9761183-2-9

Special quantity discount or sample copies for promotional sales may be available from Agilceed Books. For more information, please write to the Sales Manager, Educational Publishing, Agilceed Books at 309 Woodbine Drive, Terre Haute, IN 47803. For information on bulk purchase prices, translations or book distributors outside the U.S.A., please contact Agilceed Books at agilceed@gmail.com.

October, 2006

Acknowledgment

We would like to express our gratefulness to Mr. Shawn Waltz, a long time Tai Chi practitioner, who spent his valuable time reviewing the manuscripts of this book carefully. His valuable suggestions and corrections make this book better source of reference.

Preface

Tai Chi is the sound translation of a classic Chinese martial art. The literal meaning of Tai Chi or Tai Chi Chuan is the Grand Ultimate Fist, although rarely would people talk about Tai Chi using this term. Other spellings include Taichi, T'ai Ch'i, Tai Qi, Taiji Quan, and Tai Chi Quan. Tai Chi is one of the most celebrated Chinese Martial Arts, created and developed over thousands of years. History records show many well-known Tai Chi masters were from the Wu Dang Mountains in Hu Bei, China (the home of Taoism). Tai Chi has solid philosophical and martial art foundations. It is distinctive from other martial arts in its theory, which says that the soft is hard and will break the hard. Tai Chi appears slow and yielding but it has great power hidden underneath. This is what Tai Chi masters described as "the needle hidden in the cotton," which is the secret that allows the weakest to overcome the strongest. In the last hundred years, Tai Chi has evolved to be a great form of fitness and heath exercise for average people rather than being studied for combat purpose only.

The sword is the most widespread weapon around the globe, but varies greatly in size and shape. The Tai Chi sword is very popular in China. It is lightweight and narrow in shape. In Tai Chi principle the agility and softness will overcome the brutal force. So an agile wielding of sword is suitable for Tai Chi moves. For fitness exercise, a very light sword is very easy to use and a 90-year old Chinese will still be able to use it well.

In this book, we will introduce the 32 simplified forms of Tai Chi Sword in four groups. Each form will be described in detail as well as the keys to performing it. This book is a good source of reference. However, for students who just begin learning Tai Chi

Sword, a person-to-person learning in a class form is recommended. It is important to find a good teacher. Without a qualified teacher, many students would be left with questions and guesses which could result in misunderstandings and mistakes in difficult sword forms.

Experiences tell us that the first challenge is to perform the sword forms correctly. Rarely are books enough for showing the sequences of Tai Chi moves and the subtleness of turns. To aid the learning process, we made a separate DVD video to show how the sword forms were performed. The DVD presents Tai Chi Sword forms in the same order as in this book. The purpose is to make the learning process easy and fun to follow. It is recommended that students learn Tai Chi Sword after at least one year of practices of Tai Chi Chuan. Some masters may require students to learn Tai Chi Sword after 3 years of the hand form training. It is hoped that this book and the DVD will provide enough information for a beginner to get started, and at the same time serve as a good source of reference for the experienced Tai Chi Sword enthusiast.

Don Zhao
October 10, 2006

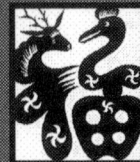

Table of Contents

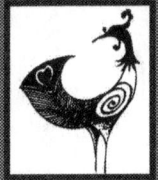

TABLE OF THE 32 FORMS

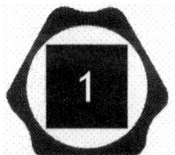

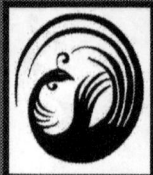

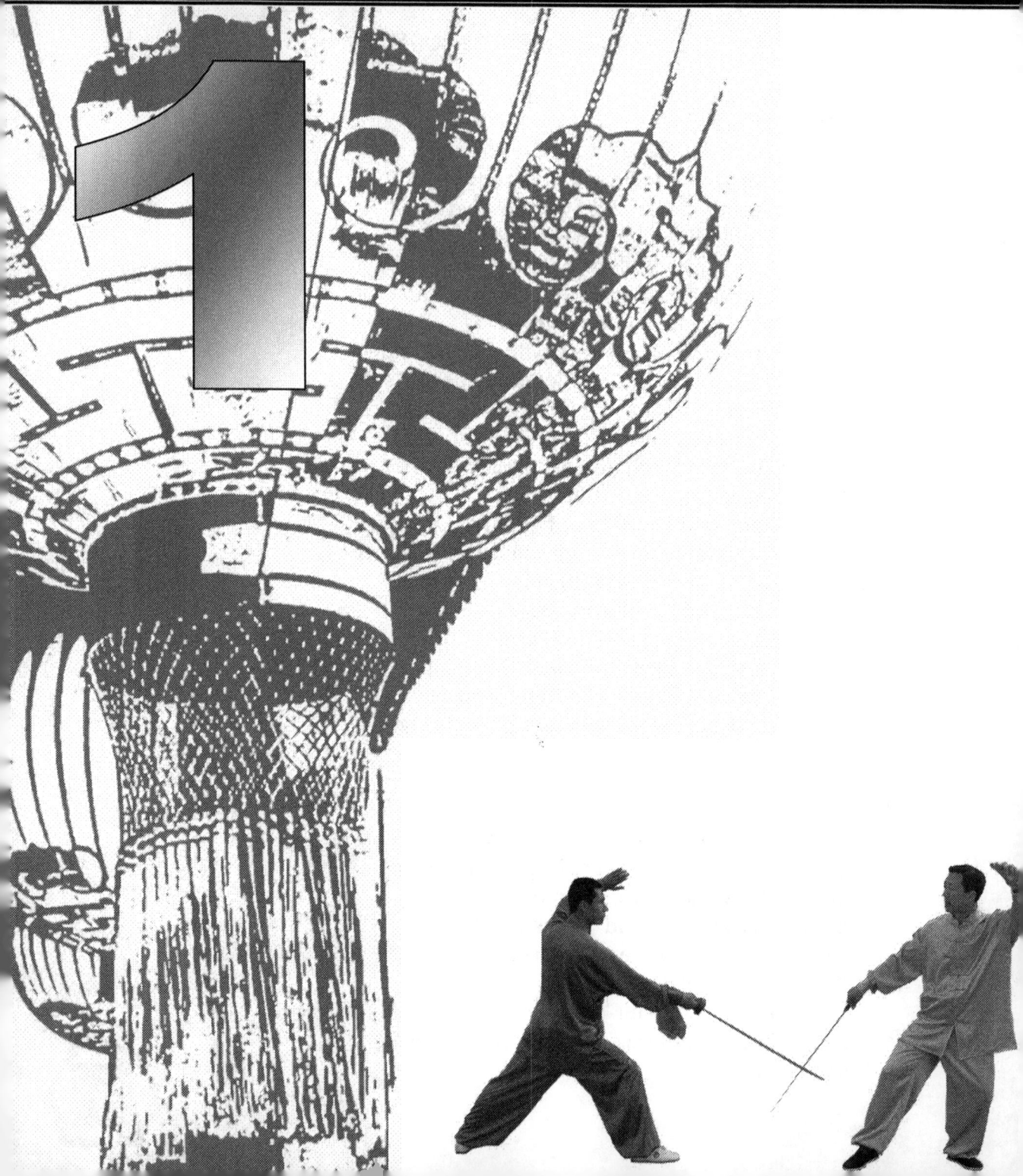

1

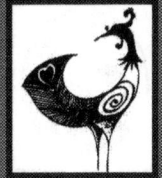

Chapter 1: Introduction

Brief History

Tai Chi Sword is a weaponry form of Tai Chi practice, in which the sword is viewed as an extension of body, not a separate part of Tai Chi practice. All Tai Chi weaponry forms preserve the same principles of Tai Chi Chuan (the hand form of Tai Chi). It is believed that everyone shall first learn Tai Chi Chuan well before starting to learn any weaponry form of Tai Chi. Other Tai Chi weapons include broadsword, spear and staff. The 32 simplified forms described in this book are the standard practice form of Tai Chi Sword created by the Chinese Sports Committee in 1957. In this form, Yang style of Tai Chi Sword was chosen because of its popularity and simplicity. The Yang style Tai Chi was formed by three generations of Yang family Tai Chi masters over more than one hundred years (1799 – 1936).

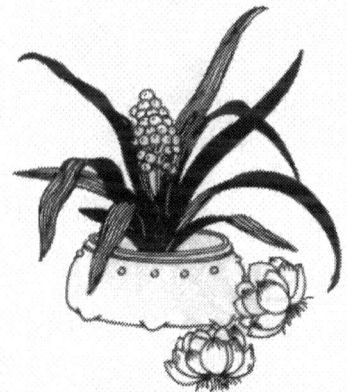

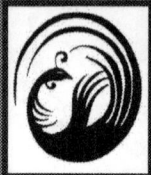

Yang Lu Chan (1799 – 1872), a disciple of Chen Chang Xing, first created a Tai Chi style of his own after many years of training with Chen. He came to Beijing to teach Tai Chi Chuan in 1820. He promoted Tai Chi as a way of improving health and fitness instead of a pure form of martial art. After his modifications of Tai Chi forms, difficult moves and postures that require big jumps and Qi power were removed. Yang Lu Chan formed a distinctive style of Tai Chi that is graceful and smooth flowing in its practice. It is called small frame Tai Chi. His third son Yang Jian Hou (1839 – 1917) and his grandson Yang Cheng Pu (1883 – 1936) further refined the Yang style Tai Chi, which are called medium frame and big frame, respectively. After China's civil war (1945 – 1949), Tai Chi of all family styles became stabilized. More efforts were made to promote Tai Chi practice among average citizens mainly for the purpose of health benefits. This is one of the reasons that Tai Chi is now so widespread and popular among average people all over the world today.

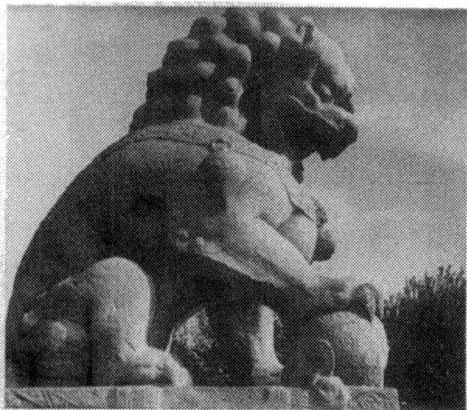

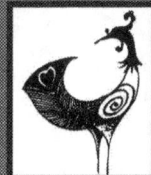

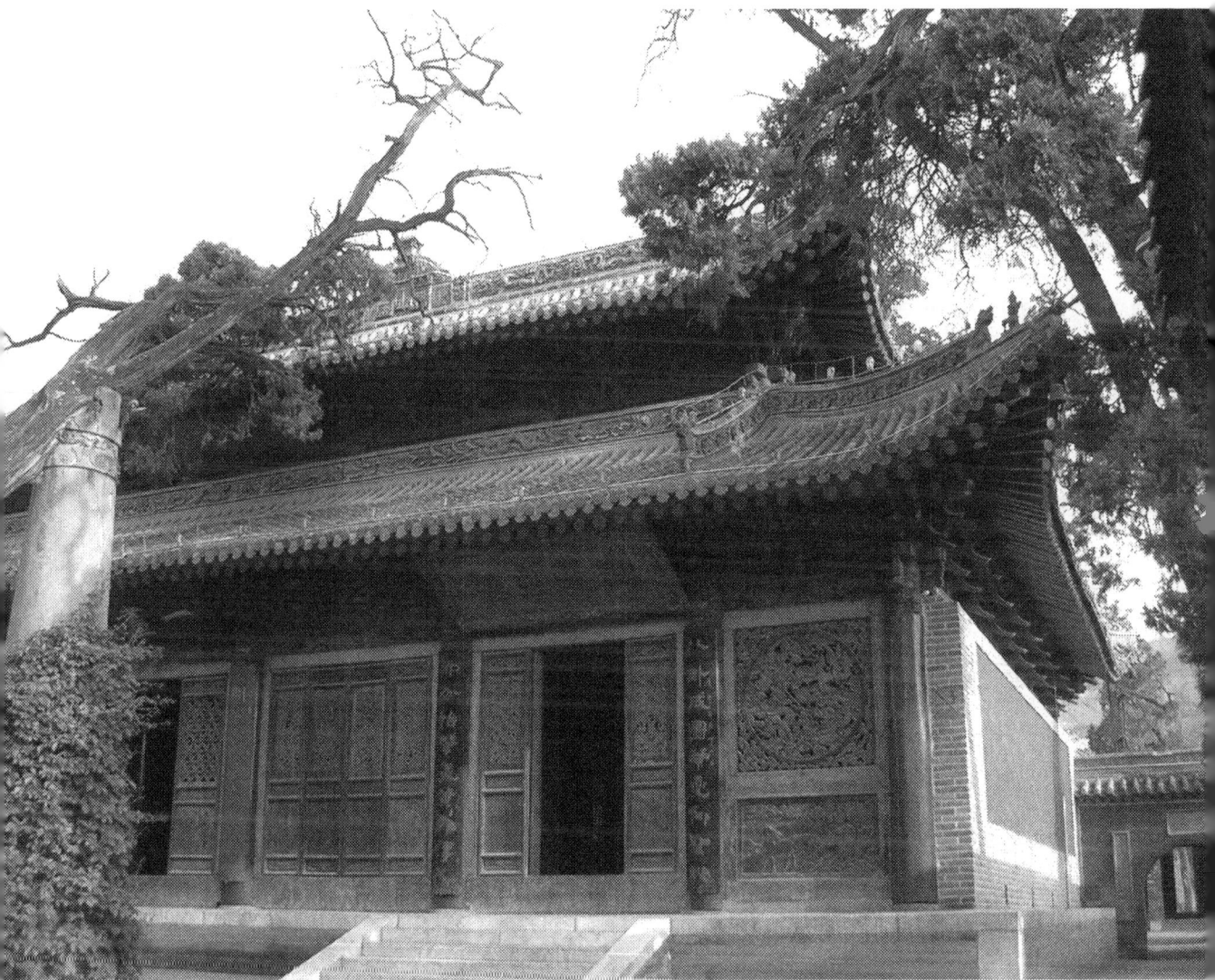

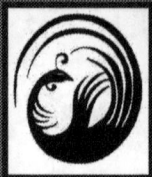

Health Benefits

Over centuries of refinement, Tai Chi Sword has evolved into a fitness exercise in the form of Chinese martial art. Although every form of Tai Chi Sword can be practiced for real martial combat, most people now choose to have a lightweight or even a wood sword in their daily practice for the purpose of improving fitness. Interestingly, there are two versions of form names of Tai Chi sword. One version is succinct description of physical moves that bear combat meanings and the other has been beautified with poetic descriptions of nature and animals, which is in the true taste of Taoism – the spirit of natural forces. Tai Chi Sword follows the philosophy of Taoism and uses it as the spirit of practice. . The spirit is more important than the force and agility of a fight. More importantly, the intent is to improve health and to wave sword as a mind-body exercise. Together, Tai Chi Sword is a supreme method for improving mental and physical health.

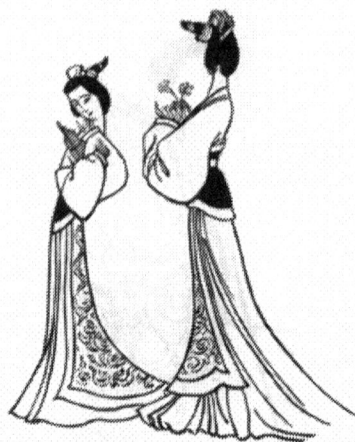

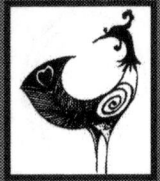

Ancient in its origin and deep in spiritual roots, Tai Chi Sword is "moving meditation" that unifies body and mind, the same way as the interaction of yin and yang. The sword is light and agile and its movements are graceful and slow, soft and coordinated, continuous and flowing, relaxed and dynamic. The goal is to harmonize the body, mind, and spirit for the greatest health benefits.

As a healing art, Tai Chi helps control a wide range of common chronic ailments such as arthritis, high blood pressure, and heart and respiratory problems. It is also effective in:

- Enhancing sensory awareness
- Improving flexibility, coordination, and concentration
- Increasing physical strength and stamina
- Improving concentration and memory
- Regulating bodily organs naturally
- Relieving stress and pain

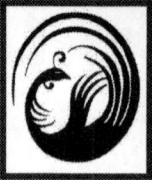

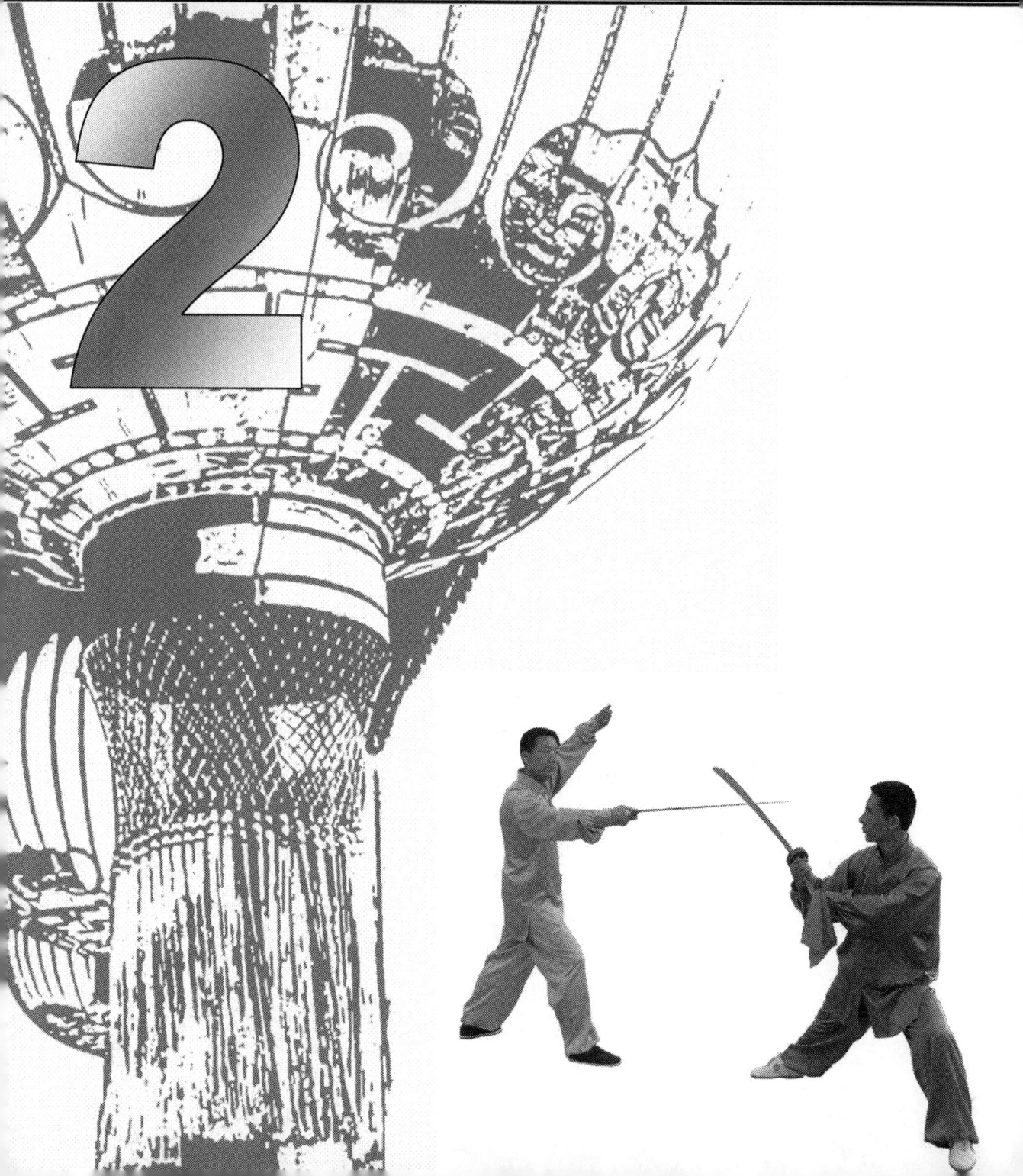

2

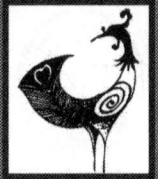

Chapter 2: Learning the Sword

Shapes and Sizes of Sword

Traditionally, the Tai Chi Sword was crafted based upon the preference of the user. The size and habits of the user were taken into account since the sword is supposed to be an integral part of the martial artist of Tai Chi. In general, a Tai Chi sword is about 3 feet in length and 2 – 3 inches in width. The sword is double edged with the blade running from the tip of the sword to almost the top of the handle portion. The blade is about 2.5 feet. As to the use of sword, the blade has three areas for different functions: (1) the tip is razor sharp and the upper third is sharpened for slashing. Since this area is easily broken, it is not for blocking. Instead, it is for pointing and piercing; (2) the middle area of the blade is still sharp but thicker than the tip. This area is used for cutting and chopping and directing away the

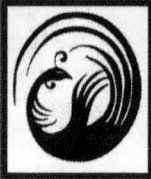

attacking weapon; (3) the third area is near the hilt. It is structurally the strongest part of blade. When meeting with brutal and violent power, it was used to block or shove away the opponent. The handle or the hilt is about 8 inches. At the end of the hilt, often there is a round hole for tying a decorative knot or a tassel.

Modern Tai Chi swords are mass-produced. They are a lot lighter than traditional ones and made of thin alloy or wood. The swords have weaponry forms, but are non-functional. They are dull and lightweight for daily exercise or competitions at martial art tournaments. These Tai Chi swords are narrower than traditional ones, about 3 feet in length and 2 inches in width. The tips are rounded and the swords have no blade at all.

Basic Techniques

- There are basic techniques in Tai Chi sword practice as to how to hold the sword, how the eyes look and follow the sword, and how the body moves. These techniques also explain how to step and use legs. Of course, the ways

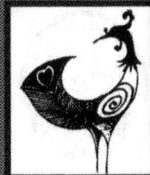

of using the sword are the most important part of all.

- sword holding methods include: (1) Flat Holding, (2) Straight Holding, (3) Pliers Holding, (4) Carrying Holding, (5) Opposite Holding and (6) Back-Handed Holding;
- Eye looking methods include: (1) Looking Flat to the Front, and (2) Eyes Following Sword;
- Step patterns include: (1) T-stance, (2) Bow Stance, (3) Close Steps, (4) Crouch Down, (5) One-leg Stand, (6) Empty Step, (7) Horse Stance, and (8) Resting Stance;
- Stepping methods include: (1) Step Forward, (2) Retreat Step, (3) Jump and (4) Follow step
- Foot methods include: (1) Kick, (2) Part Steps, (3) Raising the Rear Leg, (3) Sweeping Leg, (4) Front Kick, (5) Balance.

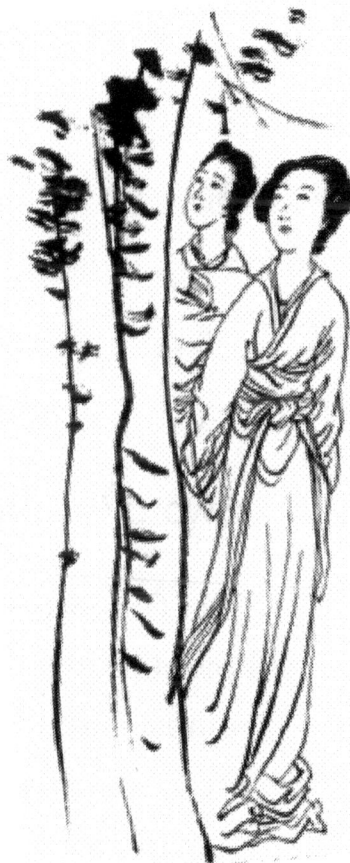

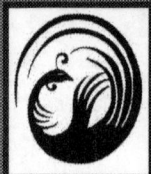

Tai Chi sword has thirteen fundamental weapon movements, which are: lashing, carrying, raising, blocking, striking, piercing, pointing, felling, stirring, pressing, chopping, intercepting and clearing. Knowing these movements well will greatly help break down the form structure and help you understand the sword movements.

点、pointing   刺、piercing   扫、sweeping
带、lashing,   Slicing, Lead   劈、chopping   抽、
pulling   撩、swing   拦、intercepting, blocking
挂、hang up   托、raising, holding up   截、Cutting,
Intercept   击、striking,   抹、Wipe around

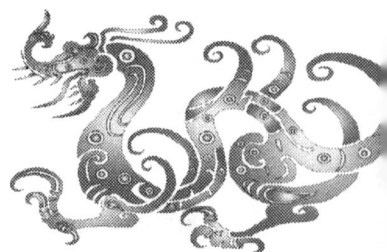

Sword Framework

Tai Chi Sword is an important part of overall Tai Chi practice, which has the style and characteristics of both empty-hand Tai Chi forms and swordsmanship. The practice of Tai Chi sword requires a person to follow the sword forms correctly, to balance the sword well with the body and to apply power to the right of point of force. It also requires the person to understand and display as well

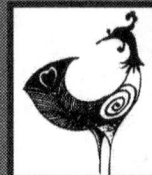

the meanings of offensive and defensive moves within each form. It is important to show accurately the shift of body weight, the empty (insubstantial) and solid (substantial) moves, and the variations of sword forms. The ultimate goal is to move the body and sword in unity with the right balance and rhythm.

Today's Tai Chi Sword has shifted its focus to the health and fitness part of the Tai Chi practice. However, as Peter Lim said: "It consists of both civil and martial portions. One without the other is incomplete". The martial or combat aspects together with combat principles and applications are still the soul of Tai Chi moves. Without understanding of the offensive and defensive meanings, the Tai Chi practice will eventually become a dance, not Tai Chi itself.

If you are a beginner, you shall start with mimicking the forms of Tai Chi sword. It is sometimes call the framework of Tai Chi. Learning the framework means that you find a teacher or take a book like this one and learn the names and movements of the forms of Tai Chi Sword one by one. It is important to learn to perform each form correctly.

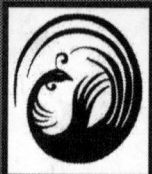

You should find a quiet place and let you body and mind be at peace before you start. This way you will have your mind concentrate on the movements of forms and think over each form you have learned. Compare what you learn with the book and find the differences as soon as they occur. Correct the mistakes at the very beginning and do not let the incorrect form set in your mind. Otherwise it will be impossible to correct later. Once you have learned the forms correctly and practiced more, you are able to understand the true meanings of Tai Chi and the inner power it gives you. In the following Chapter, we will explain the forms one by one and get you started building your framework of Tai Chi Sword.

The Form Names

The 32 forms of Tai Chi Sword are usually organized in four groups for the ease of teaching and learning. The entire form sequence starts with preparation and starting forms which are not deemed as the sword form proper; this is also true for the conclusion form. This is different from the way the 24 forms of Tai Chi Chuan are organized.

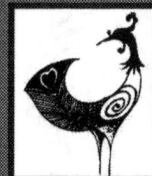

三十二式太极剑 (Tai Chi Sword)

预备式	Preparation
起势	Starting Form

第一组 Group One

1, 并步点剑	1. Point Sword with Closing Steps
2, 独立反刺	2. Opposite Pierce with One-leg Stand
3, 仆步横扫	3. Crouch Down and Sweep Sword
4, 向右平带	4. Right Slice with Bow Stance
5, 向左平带	5. Left Slice with Bow Stance
6, 独立抡劈	6. Wheel Chop Sword with One-leg Stand
7, 退步回抽	7. Step Back and Pull Sword
8, 独立上刺	8. Upward Pierce Sword with One-leg Stand

第二组 Group Two

9, 虚步下截	9. Empty Stance and Slice Downward
10, 左弓步刺	10. Pierce with Left Bow Stance
11, 转身斜带	11. Pull-back Turn and Skew Slice Sword
12, 缩身斜带	12. Contract Body and Skew Slice Sword
13, 提膝捧剑	13. Raise Knee and Hold Sword
14, 跳步平刺	14. Jump and Flat Pierce Forward
15, 左虚步撩	15. Swing Sword with Left Empty Bow Stance
16, 右弓步撩	16. Swing Sword with Right Bow Stance

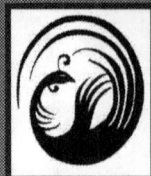

第三组 Group Three

17，转身回抽	17. Turn and Pull Sword Back
18，并步平刺	18. Close Steps and Flat Pierce
19，左弓步拦	19. Obstruct Sword with Left Bow Stance
20，右弓步拦	20. Obstruct Sword with Right Bow Stance
21，左弓步拦	21. Obstruct Sword with Left Bow Stance
22，进步反刺	22. Step Forward and Opposite Pierce
23，反身回劈	23. Reposition and Chop Back
24，虚步点剑	24. Point Sword with Empty Stance

第四组 Group Four

25，独立平托	25. Hold Sword with One-leg Up
26，弓步挂劈	26. Hang-up Chop with Right Bow Stance
27，虚步抡劈	27. Wheel Chop with Empty Stance
28，撤步反击	28. Retreat Step and Attack Backward
29，进步平刺	29. Step Forward and Flat Pierce
30，丁步回抽	30. Pull Back Sword with T-Stance
31，旋转平抹	31. Rotate and Flat Slice
32，弓步直刺	32. Forward Pierce with Left Bow Stance

收势	Conclusion

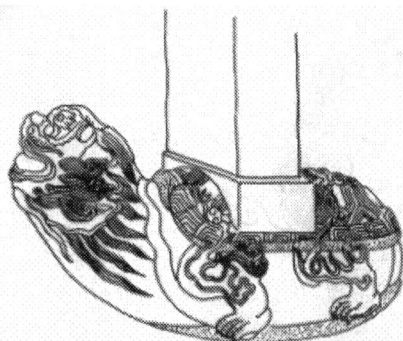

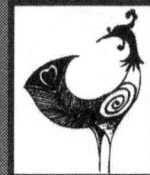

Keys to Successful Tai Chi Sword Practice

Tai Chi Sword is part of Tai Chi Chuan. The sword form was developed from the hand form. In practice, it is important to treat the body and sword as a single unit of Tai Chi movements. Tai Chi sword emphasizes the agility rather than pure force. When practicing Tai Chi, the body is flexible and the movements are agile. The circular movements shall be smooth to allow you to have perfect coordination between sword and body.

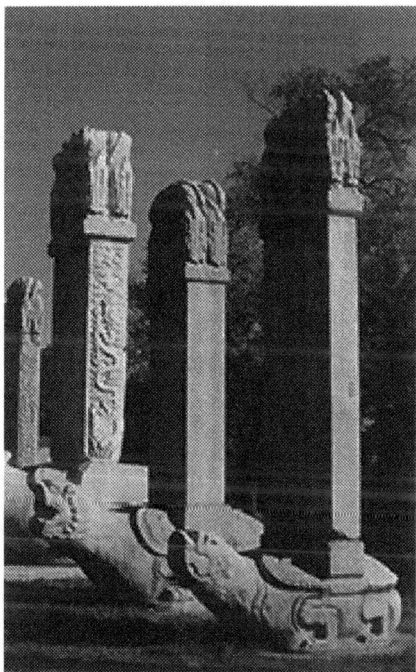

A clear and quick mind is very important in the practice Tai Chi Sword. The mind shall lead every single movement. An attentive and clear mind will make movements agile and shift well between softness and hardness. The goal is to have agile and smooth moves without rootless floating steps. Each movement shall be decisive and stable but not heavy and dragging.

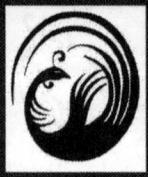

Furthermore, you shall be in high spirit and breathe naturally. The wielding of sword shall be accurate with four key characteristics: (1) touching, (2) sticking, (3) continuous, and (4) following. This is one of the reasons that some Tai Chi masters used to call the opposing practice of Tai Chi 13 Swords "the Tai Chi Sticking Sword". In sum, it is important to have mind and posture and moves to be agile and steady like swimming dragon and flying phoenix which are soft and hard with inner strength and continuous. As to the kinetics, the body movement shall be aligned to the axis of torso and move around waist. The ups and downs shall follow each other and be coordinated. The power delivered to the tip of the sword comes from the spine. The principle shall be: (1) When moving, everywhere moves; (2) When stopped, everywhere stops.

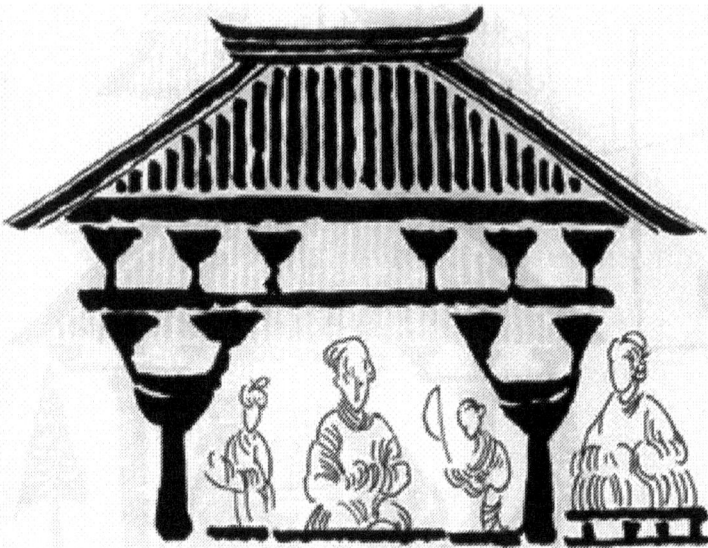

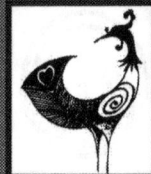

When it comes to learning the sword forms, you shall first have correct postures and forms. Secondly, practice until you are familiar with each form. This is what Tai Chi masters called "building the framework". Once you have each form learned by heart, you may take a step further to analyze the functions of each sword form. Gradually, you will be able to master the keys to using your power. This is called "practicing the framework" or touching the power. Of course, it takes an experience of competitions at tournament to step up from knowing the sword forms to knowing the power. And it takes a lot more practice for you to grow from knowing the power to sensing the divine wisdom. However, for those who practice Tai Chi Sword only for the purpose of health benefits, it is only a matter of time to achieve the level of proficiency in which it is natural to have complement of moving and stillness and interaction of the soft and the hard.

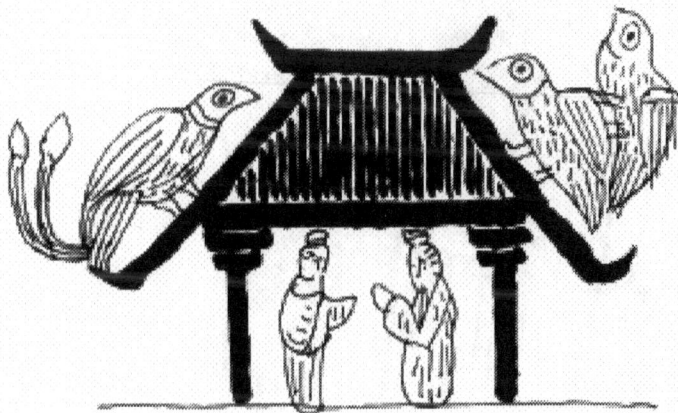

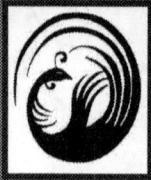

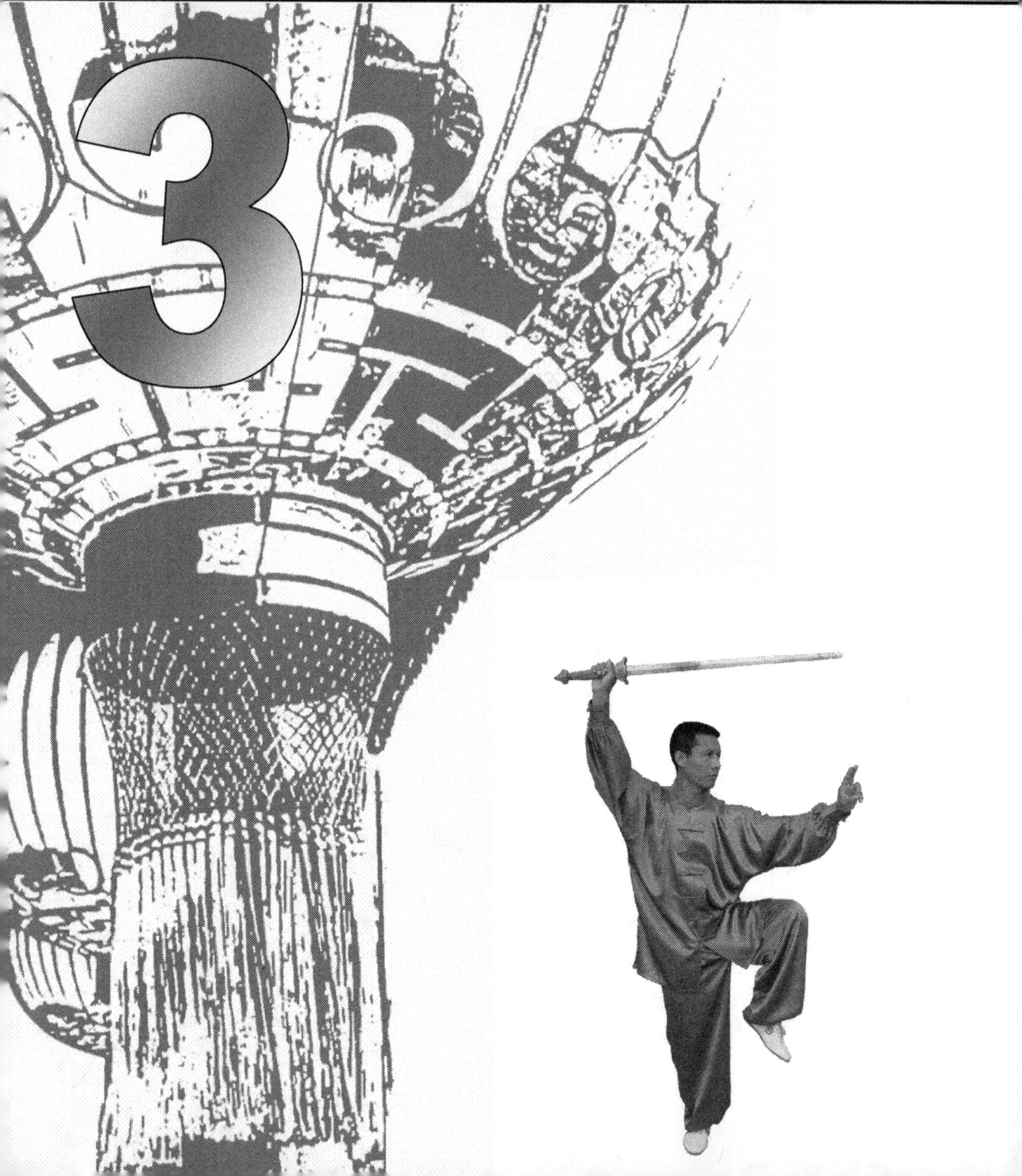

3

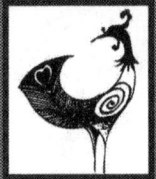

Chapter 3: The 32 Forms

The 32 sword forms follow the design of Chinese Sport Committee in 1957. The 32 forms are divided into four groups, each of which consists of eight forms. They are described as follows.

Preparation

Relax your body first, including hands, wrist, waist, ankles and all other joints.

Starting Form

The starting form or the beginning form consists of six postures. Note that this form is not a part of 32 forms listed before, although it is not any simpler than any of the 32 forms. This form gets you started from an upward standing position to a posture like drawing out your sword. That is why it is called the starting form.

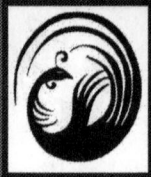

The Sequence of Beginning Form

(1) Stand naturally with both feet open to the shoulder width. Left hand holds the sword and right hand becomes a sword finger form. Sink shoulders. Look south (Figure 1).
(2) Slowly lift both arms parallel to the shoulder position. Face south (Figure 2).
(3) Rotate to the right side and circle both arms. Shift the body center to the right leg with left foot drawing close to the side of the right foot. Face south-west (Figure 3).
(4) Rotate to the left and step out left foot to left bow stance while left arm brushing the sword and right fingers pointing to the east direction. The rotation, left bow stance and both arms movements should be coordinated and soft (Figure 4).
(5) Both arms cross and rotate the body to resting stance with right arm back and left arm forward with coordination. Look west (Figure 5).
(6) Lift the left foot forward to left bow stance with both hands in front. Get ready to pass the sword from the left hand to the right hand. Face east at the end (Figure 6).

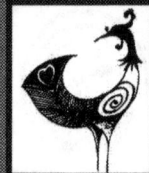

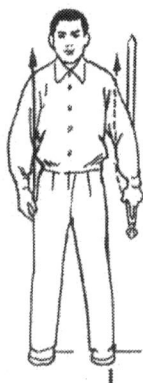

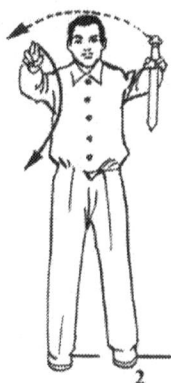

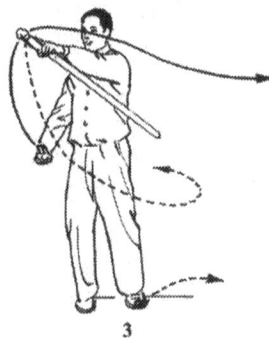

3

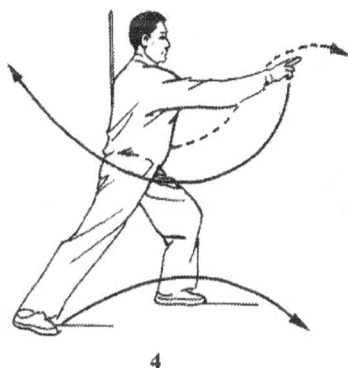

4

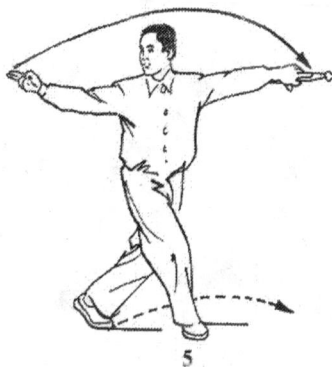

5

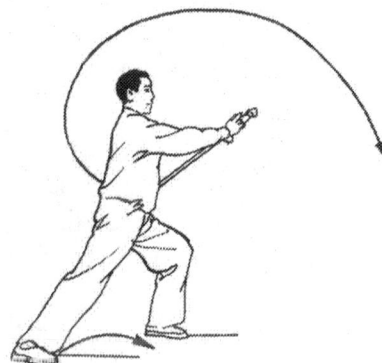

6

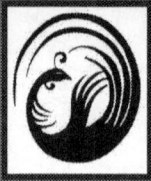

Figure 1. Stand naturally with both feet open to the shoulder width. Left hand holds the sword and right hand becomes a sword finger form. Sink shoulders. Look south.

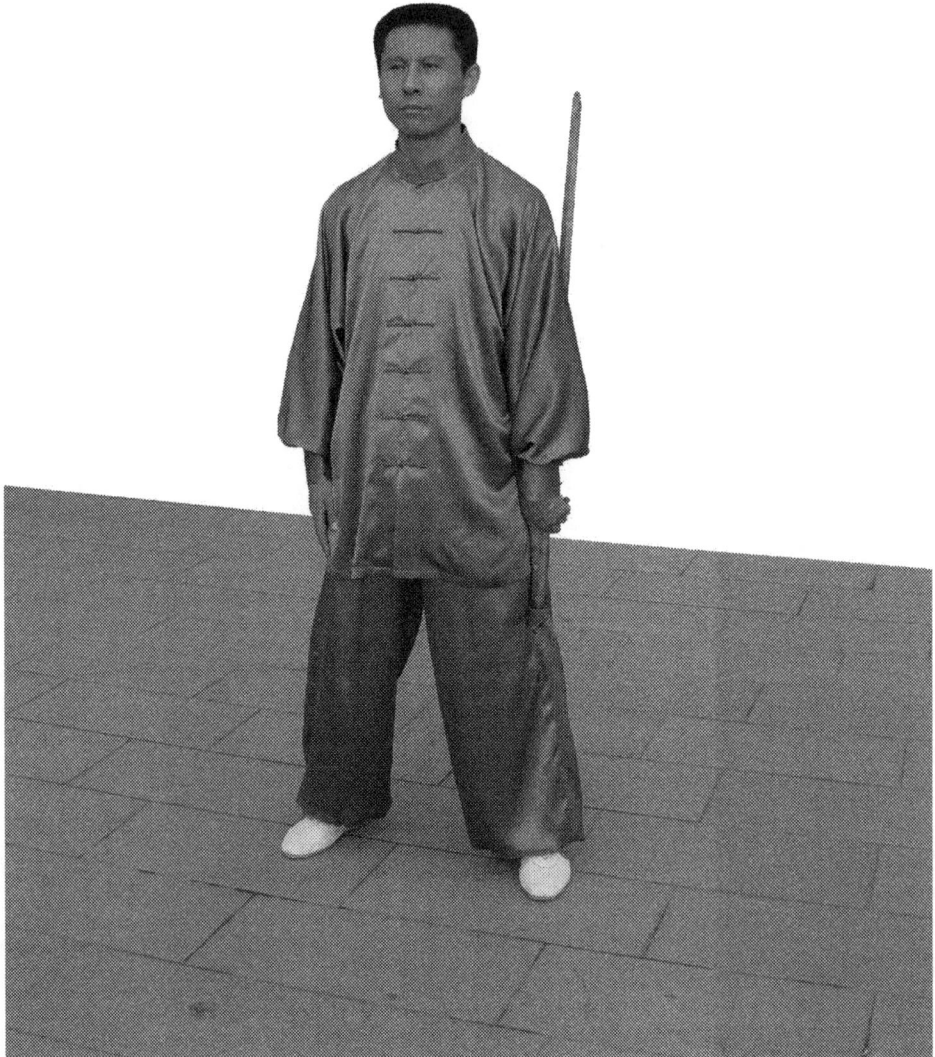

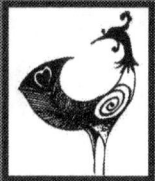

Figure 2. Slowly lift both arms parallel to the shoulder position. Face south.

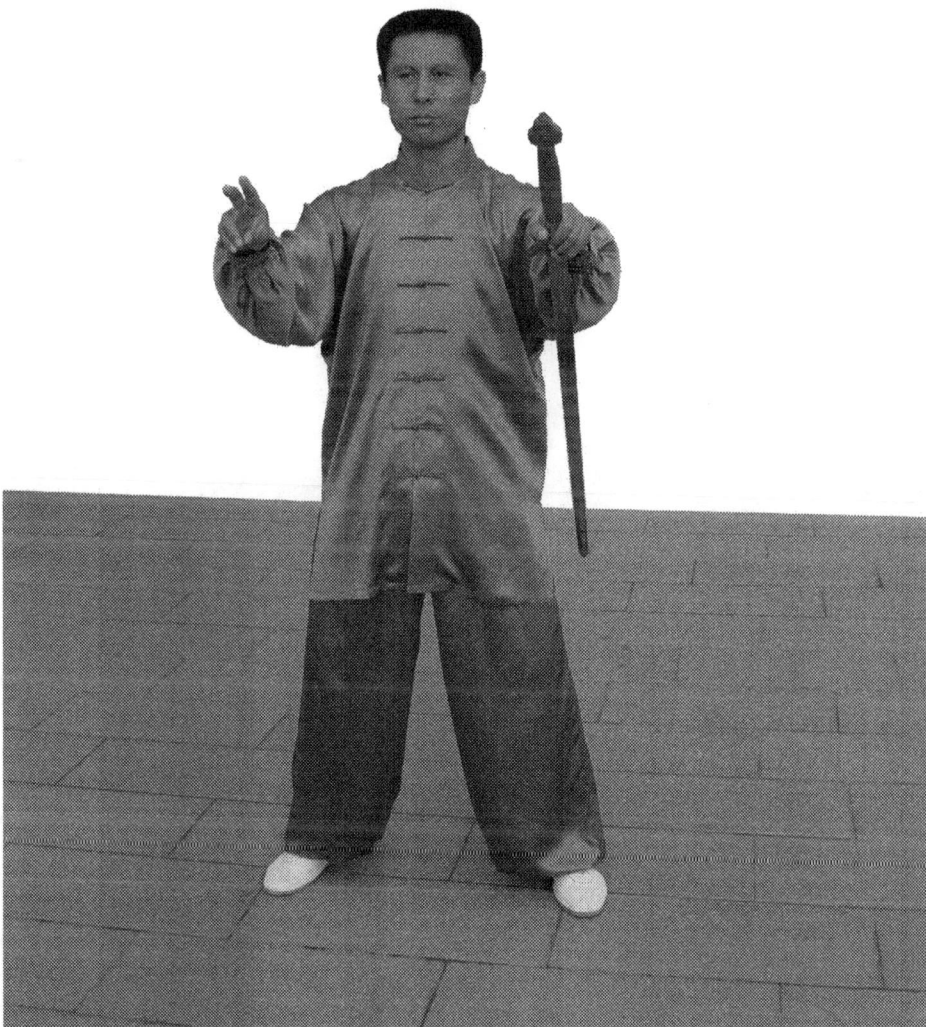

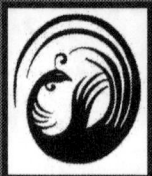

Figure 3. Rotate to the right side and circle both arms. Shift the body center to the right leg with left foot drawing close to the side of the right foot. Face south-west.

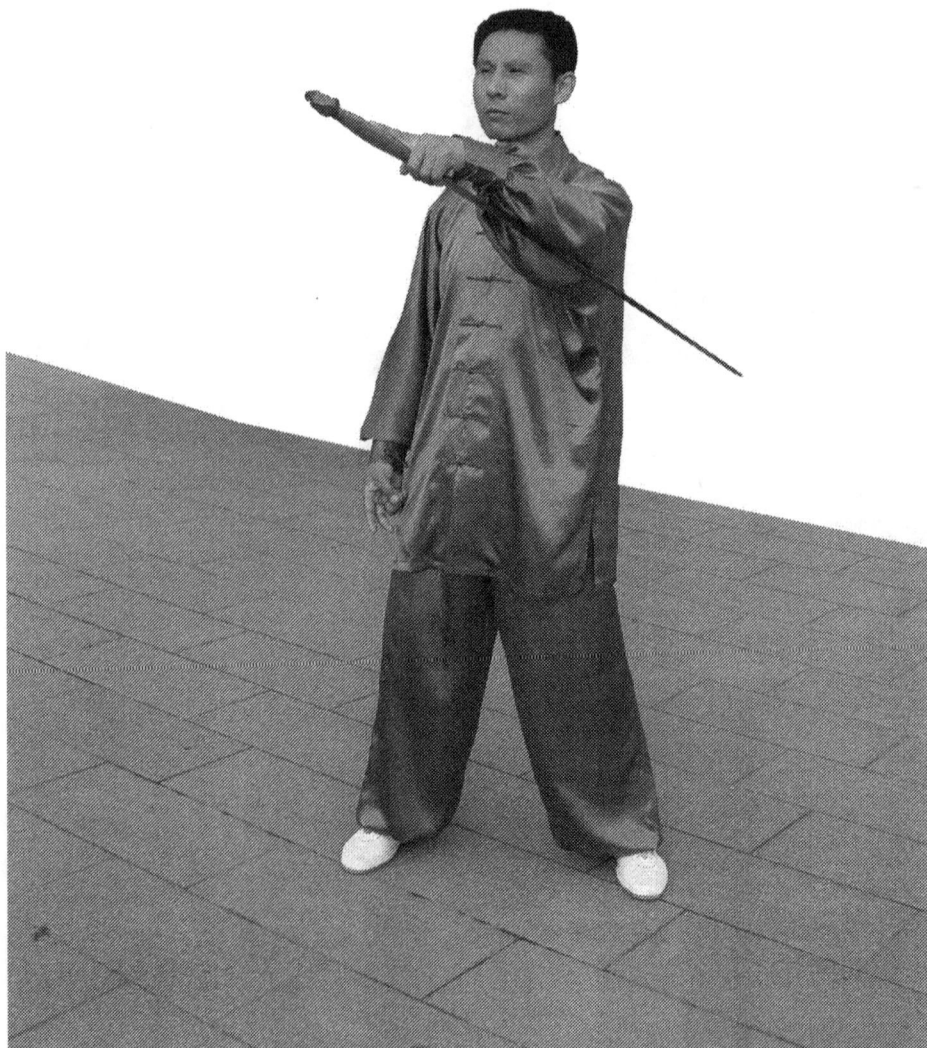

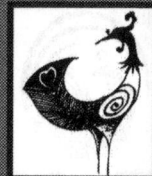

Figure 4. Rotate to the left and step out left foot to left bow stance while left arm brushing the sword and right fingers pointing to the east direction. The rotation, left bow stance and both arms movements should be coordinated and soft.

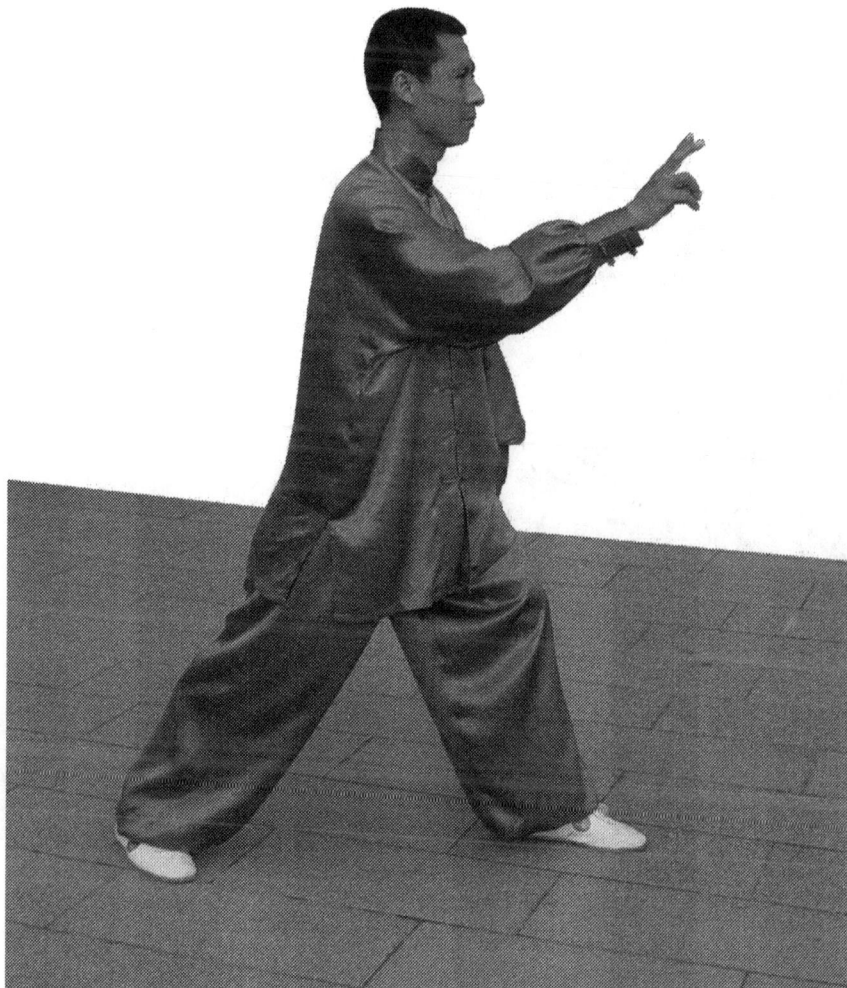

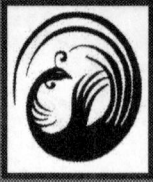

Figure 5. Both arms cross and rotate the body to resting stance with right arm back and left arm forward with coordination. Look in the west direction now.

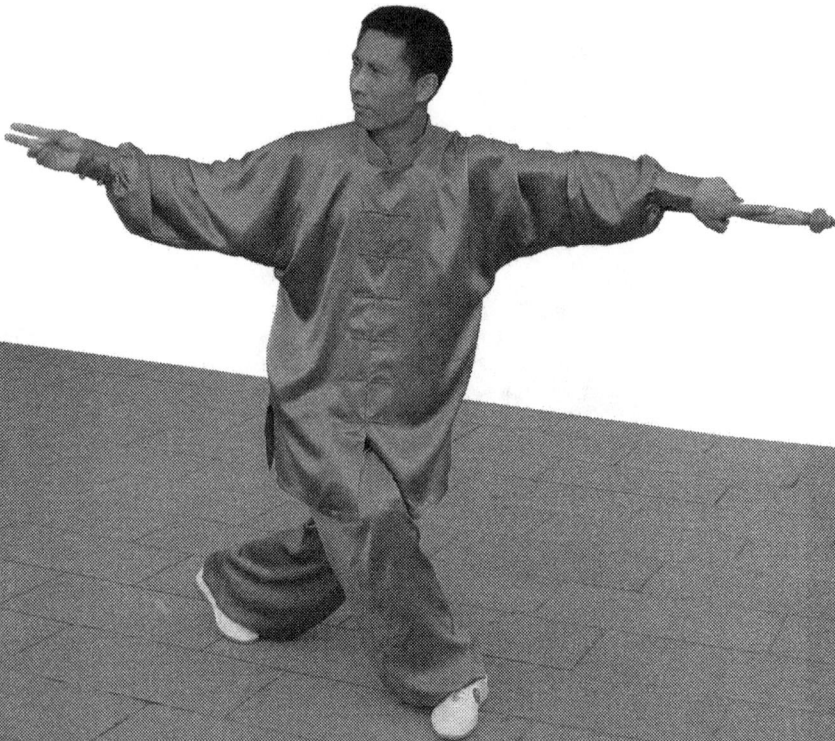

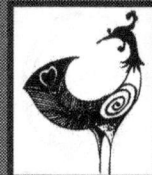

Figure 6. Lift the left foot forward to left bow stance with both hands in front. Get ready to pass the sword from the left hand to the right hand. Face east at the end.

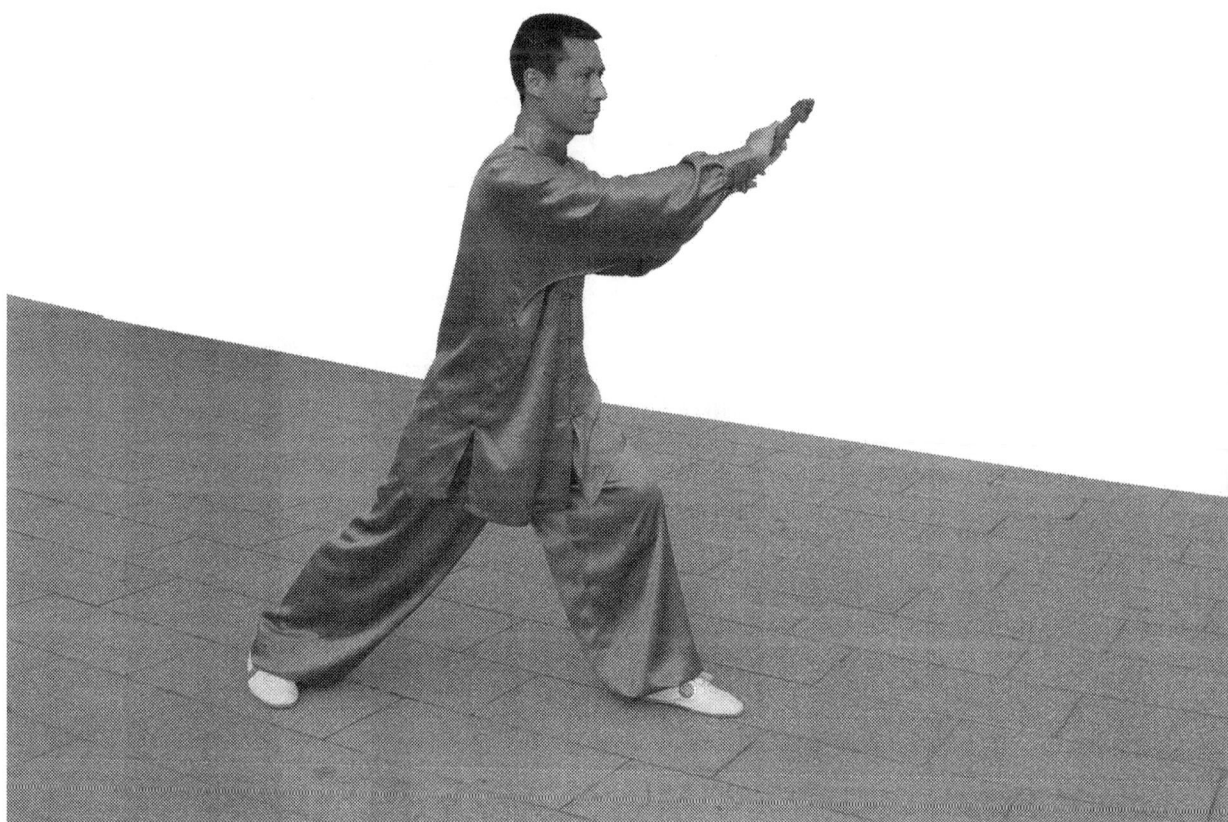

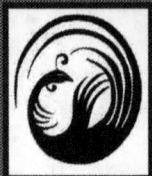

Group One

The first group consists of eight forms shown as follows.

1. *Point Sword with Closing Steps*
2. *Opposite Pierce with One-leg Stand*
3. *Crouch Down and Sweep Sword*
4. *Right Slice with Bow Stance*
5. *Left Slice with Bow Stance*
6. *Wheel Chop Sword with One-leg Stand*
7. *Step Back and Pull Sword*
8. *Upward Pierce Sword with One-leg Stand*

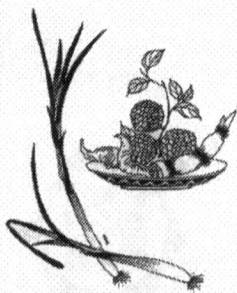

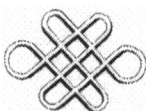

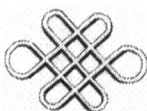

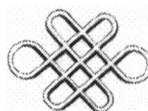

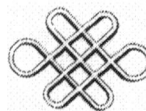

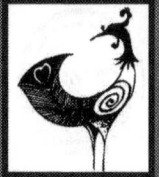

Form 1. Point Sword with Closing Steps.

(7) Pass the sword from the left hand to the right hand, vertically circle the sword to the front, and point the sword down in front, sink shoulders with upright body. Face east at the end (Figure 7).

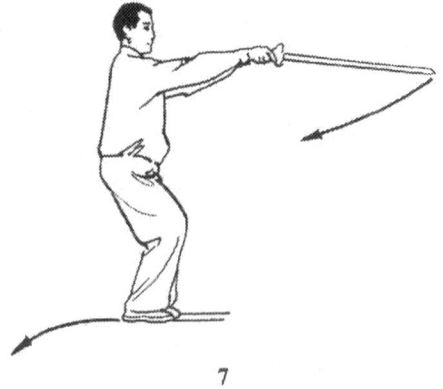

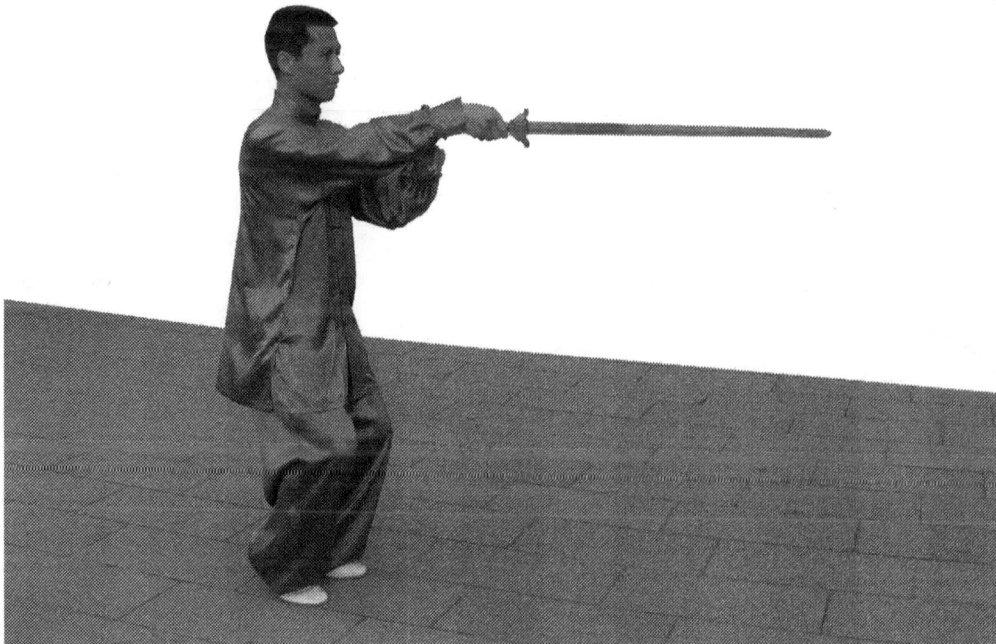

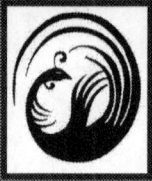

Form 2. Opposite Pierce with One-leg Stand

(8) Step back with the right foot and shift the center to the right leg while pulling the sword close to your waist (Figure 8). (9) Sit on the right leg and draw the left foot close to the right foot while circling the sword upward (Figure 9). (10) Continue to circle the sword and pierce to the east direction above your head with an independent stance standing the right leg only (Figure 10).

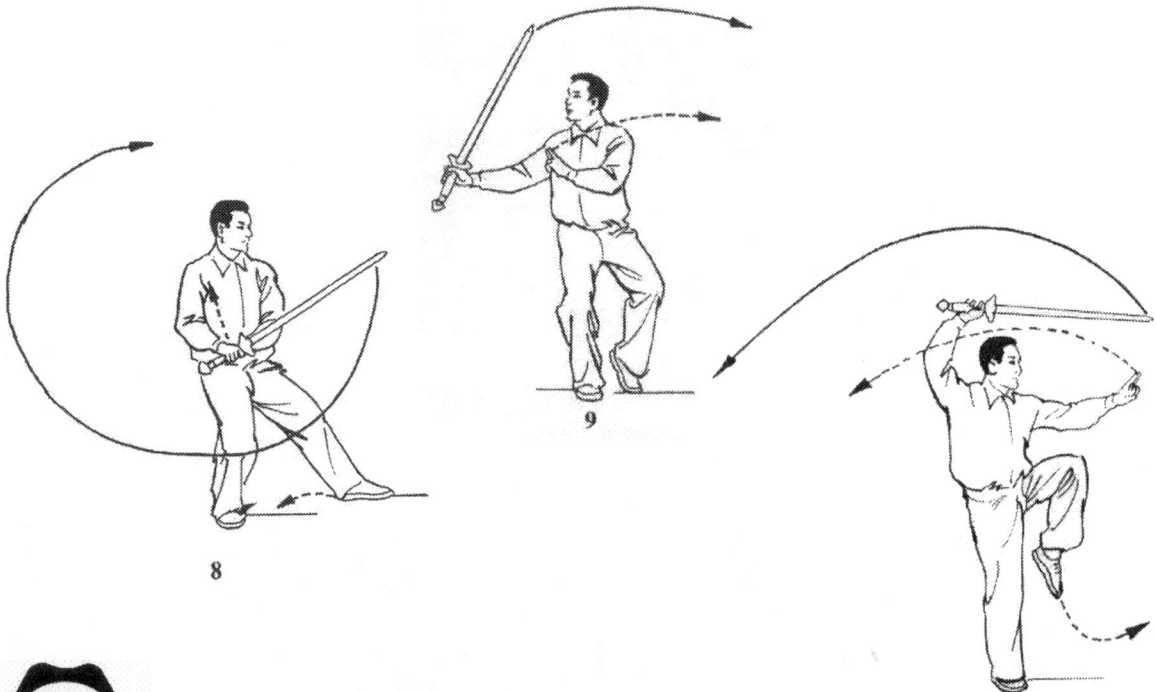

8

9

10

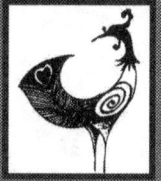

Figure 8. Step back with the right foot and shift the center to the right leg while pulling the sword close to your waist.

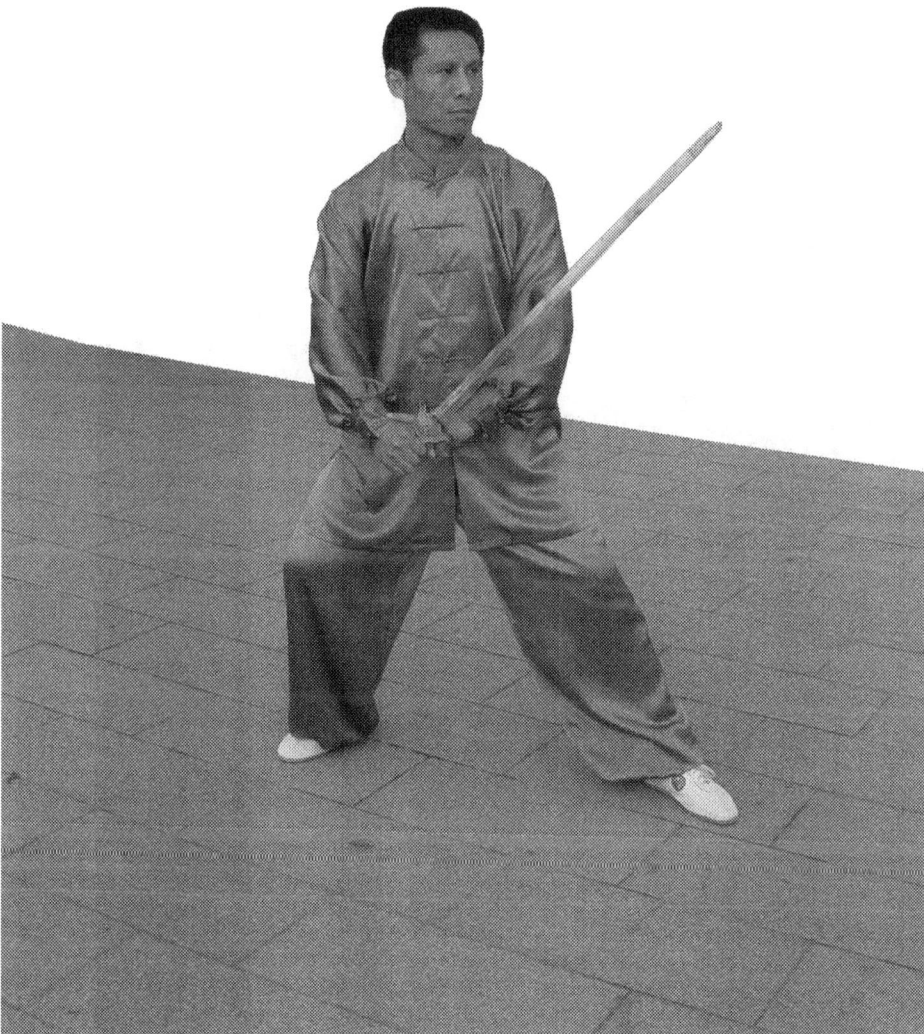

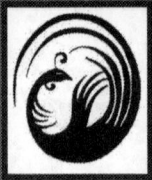

Figure 9. Sit on the right leg and draw the left foot close to the right foot while circling the sword upward.

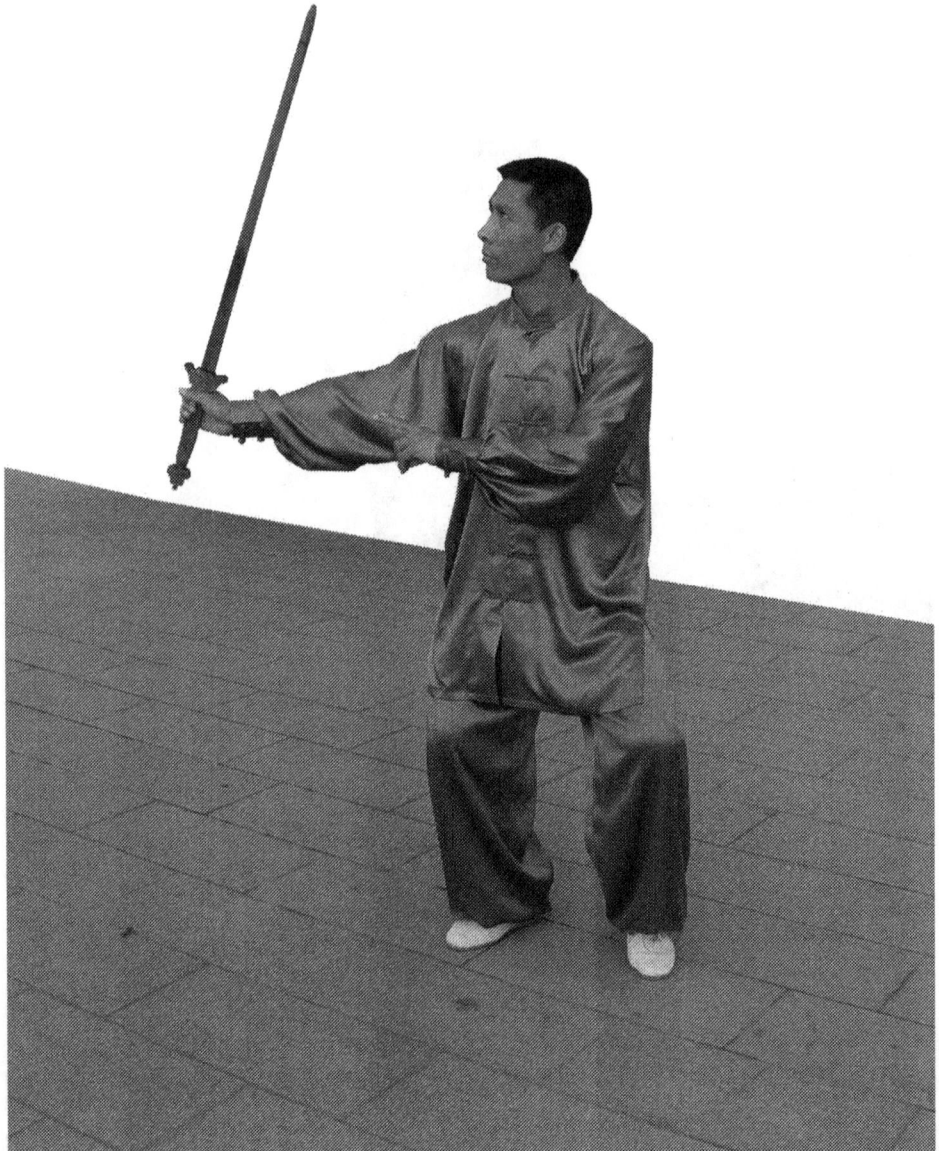

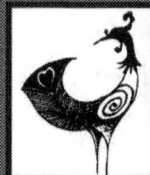

Figure 10. Continue to circle the sword and pierce to the east direction above your head with an independent stance standing on the right leg only.

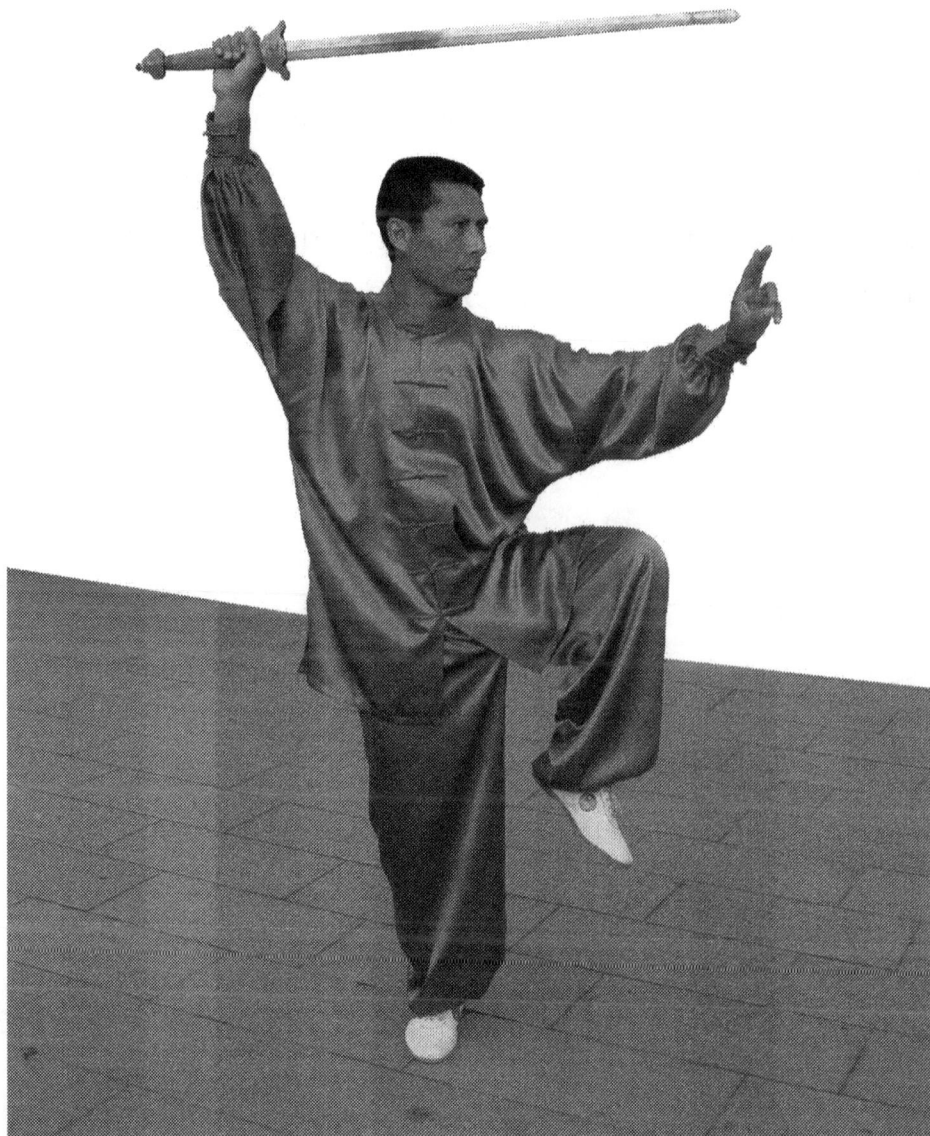

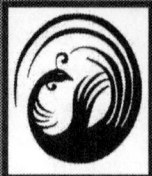
Form 3. Crouch Down and Sweep Sword

(11) Step out with the left foot forward toward northeast direction and chop the sword toward southwest direction in a right bow stance (Figure 11).

(12) Rotate the body to the left while sweeping the sword in a lower push down stance and then shift the body center from the right foot to the left foot in the left bow stance with the left arm above the head and the right hand holding the sword in front. Face east at the end (Figure 12).

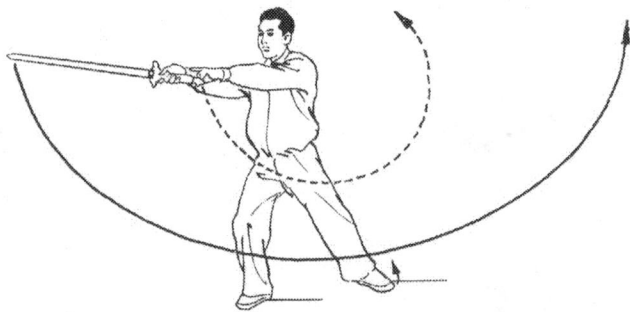

11

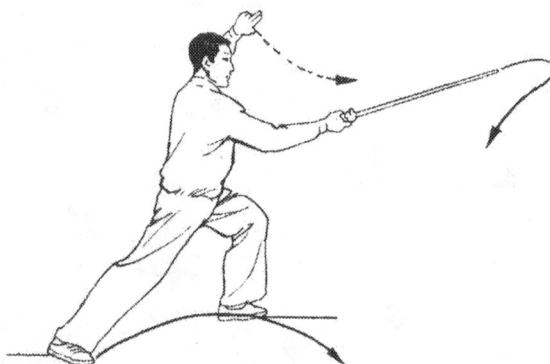

12

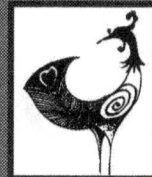

Figure 11. Step out the left foot toward northeast direction and chop the sword toward southwest direction in a right bow stance.

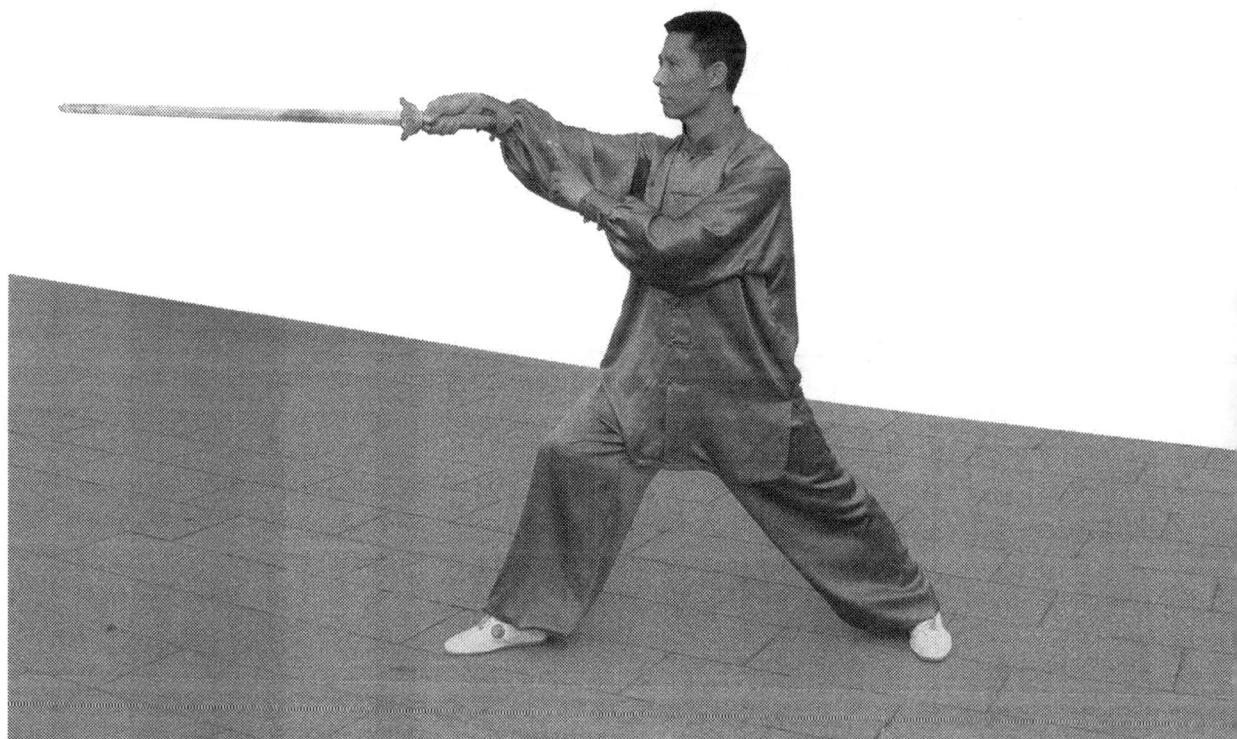

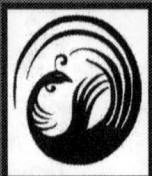

Figure 12. Rotate the body to the left while sweeping the sword in a lower push down stance and then shift the body center from the right foot to the left foot in the left bow stance with the left arm above the head and the right hand holding the sword in front. Face east at the end.

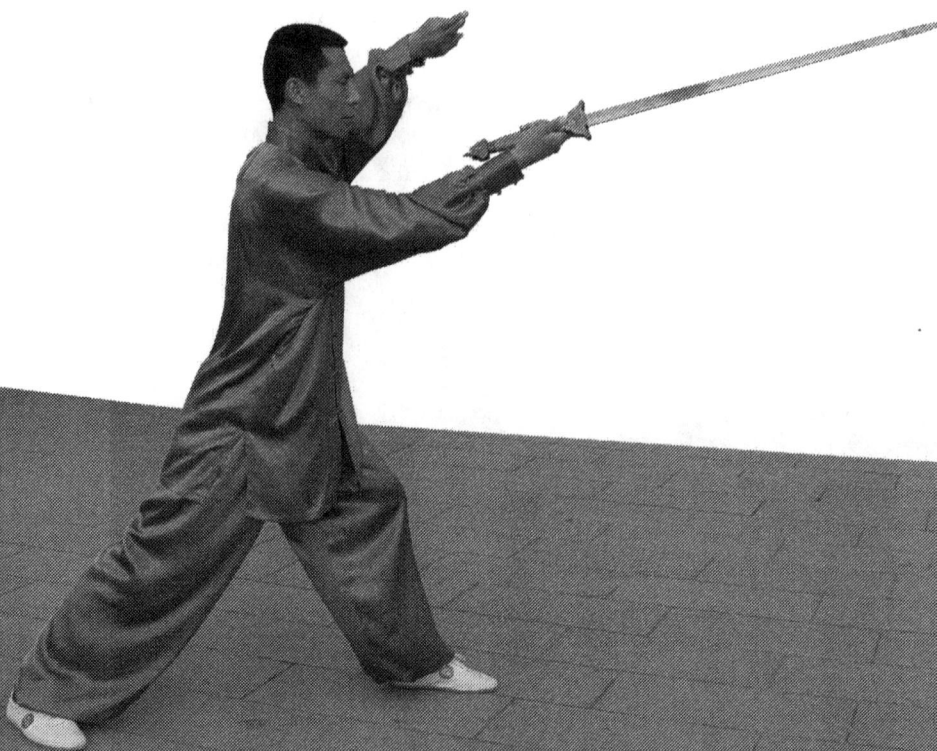

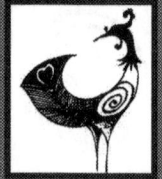

Form 4. Right Slice with Bow Stance

(13) Draw your right leg forward in a right bow stance, flip the sword, and slice the sword flatly in a curve way to the right side with the left sword fingers touching the right hand while the right hand holds the sword in front. Face east at the end (Figure 13).

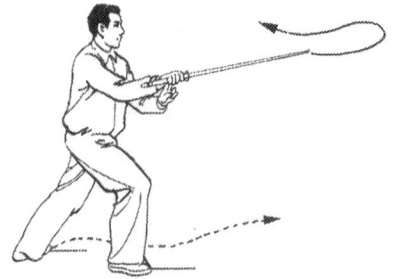

13

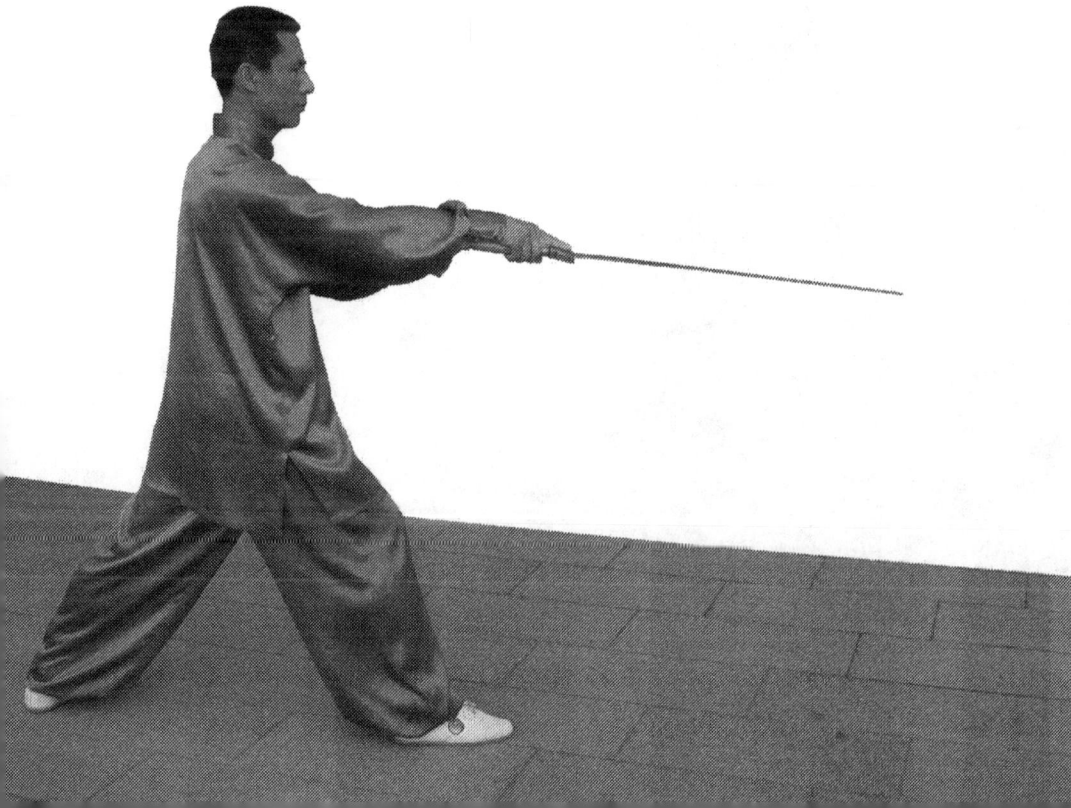

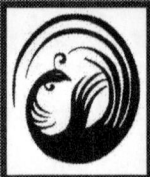

Form 5. Left Slice with Bow Stance

(14) Draw your left leg forward in a left bow stance, flip the sword and slice the sword in a curve way to the left side with the left arm above the head and the right hand holding the sword in front. Face east at the end (Figure 14).

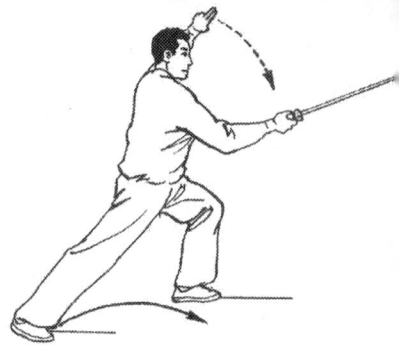

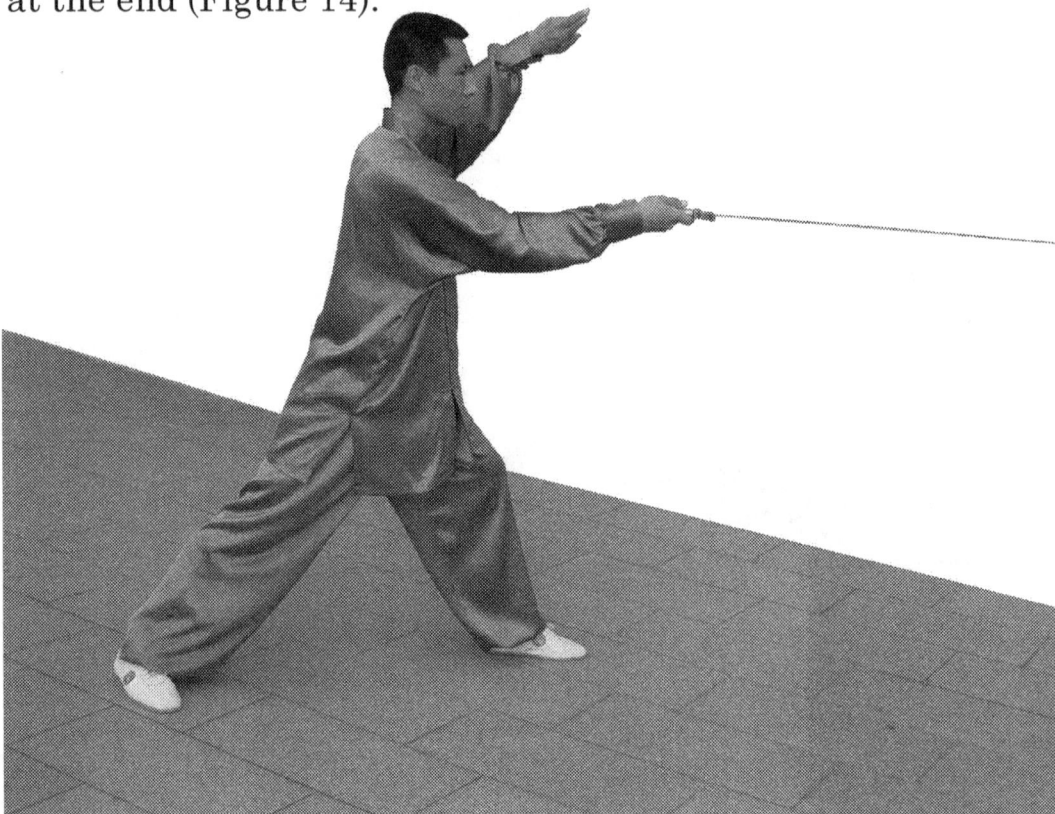

14

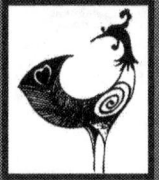

Form 6. Wheel Chop Sword with One-leg Stand

(15) Draw your right foot close to the left foot (Figure 15).
(16) Vertically circle the sword to the left side of your waist
and then to the right side (Figure 16).
(17) Step out with your right foot and then stand on the
right leg while lifting up your left leg and chop the sword in
an independent stance. Face east at the end (Figure 17).

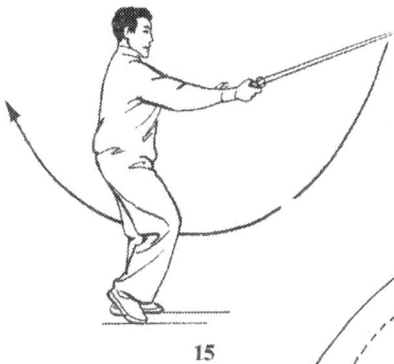

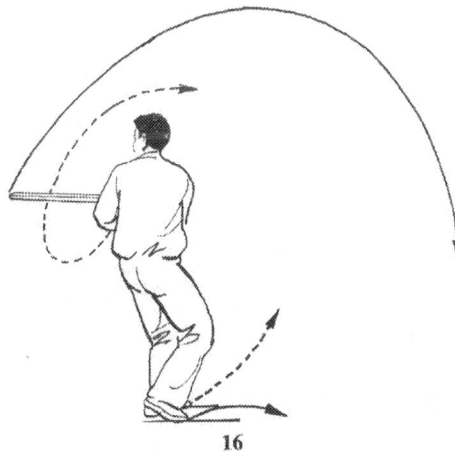

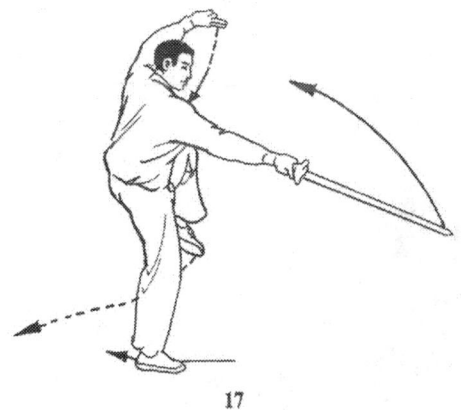

15

16

17

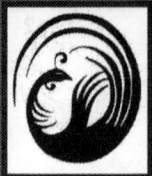

Figure 15. Draw your right foot close to the left foot.

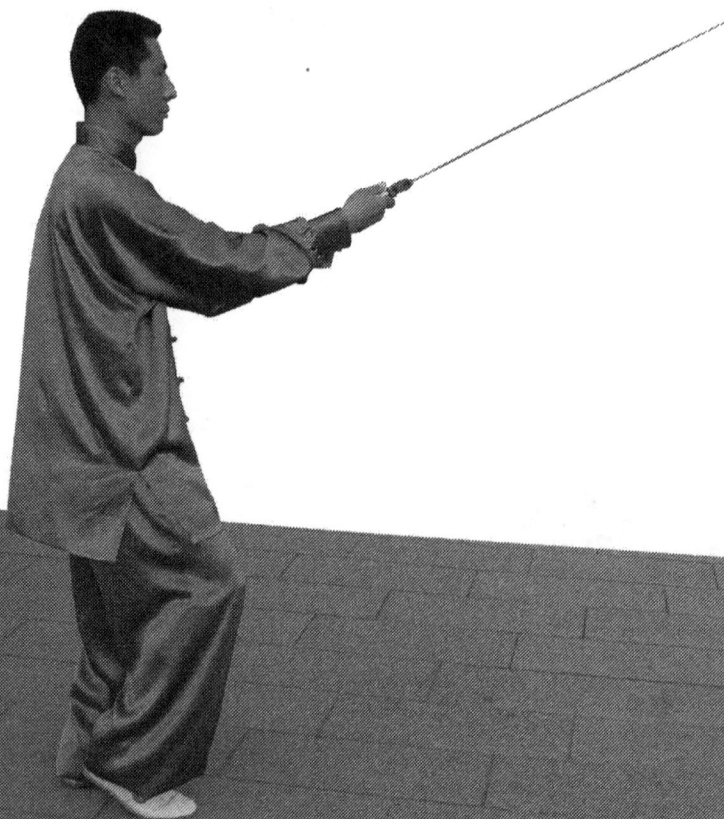

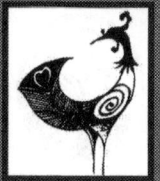

Figure 16. Vertically circle the sword to the left side of your waist and then to the right side.

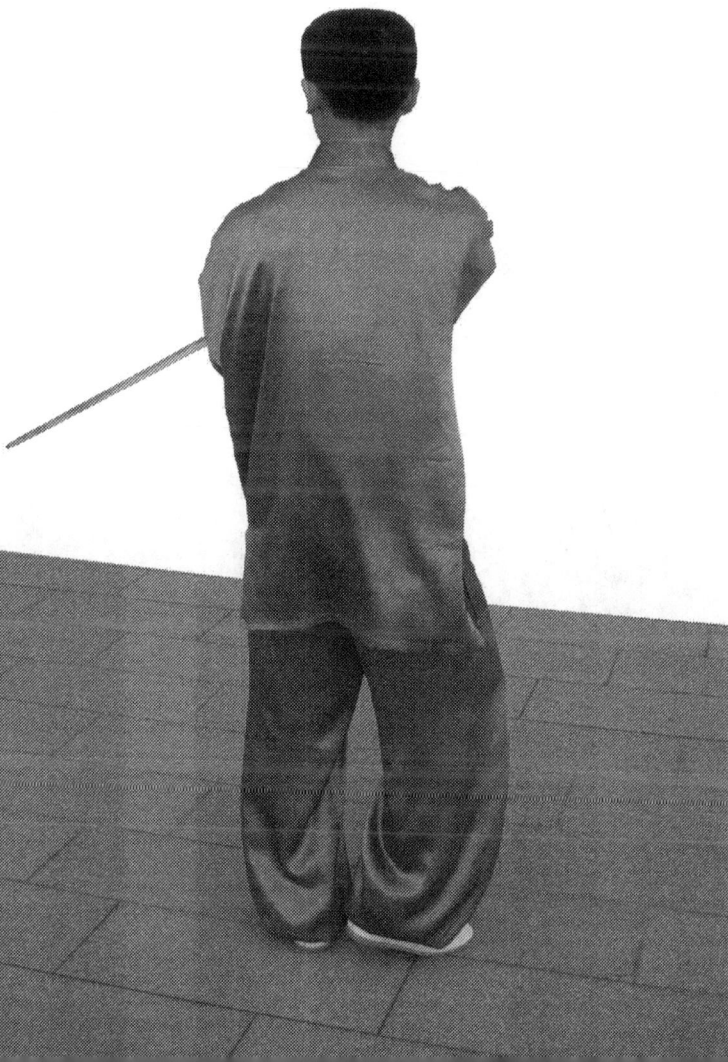

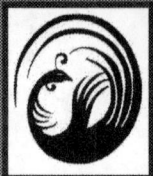

Figure 17. Step out your right foot and then stand on the right leg while lifting up your left leg, chop the sword in an independent stance. Face east at the end.

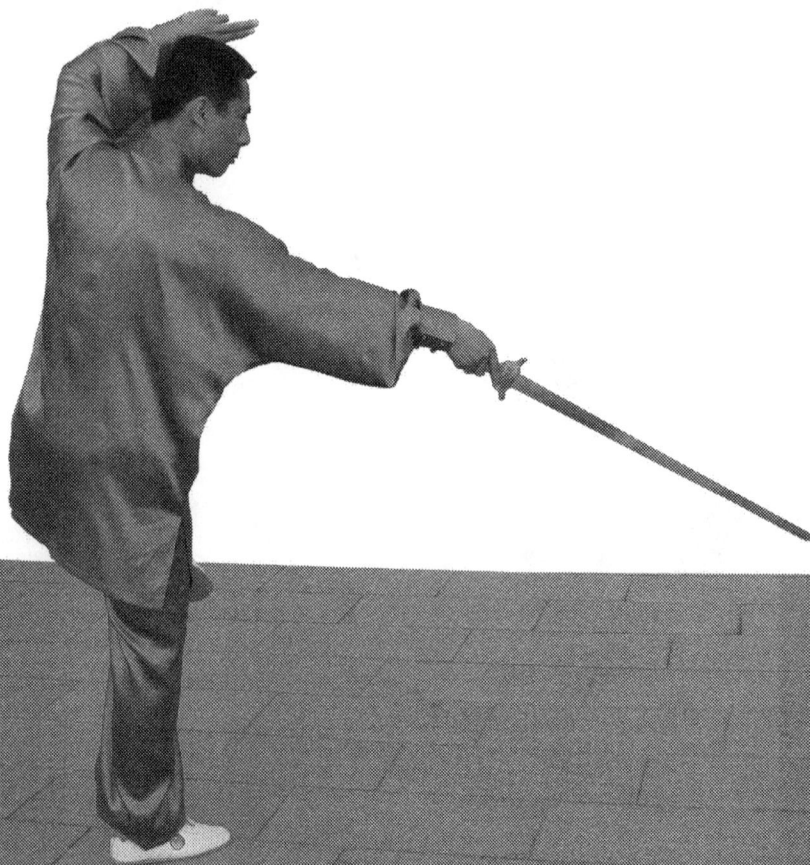

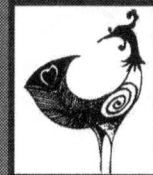

Form 7. Step Back and Pull Sword

(18) Step back in a sit on the left leg stance while pulling the sword to the chest. Face northeast (Figure 18).

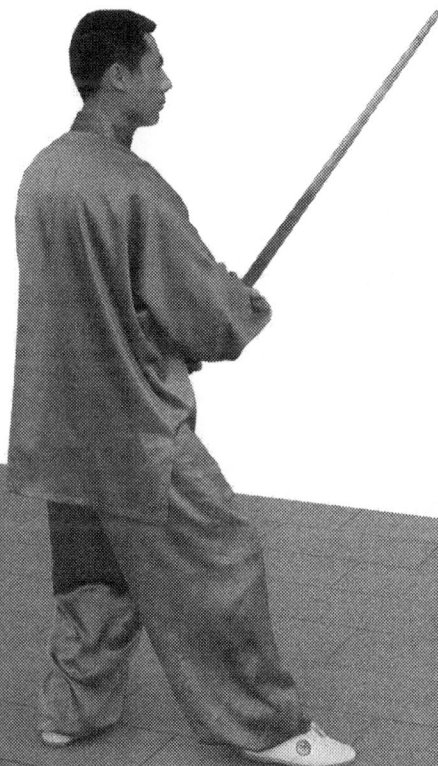

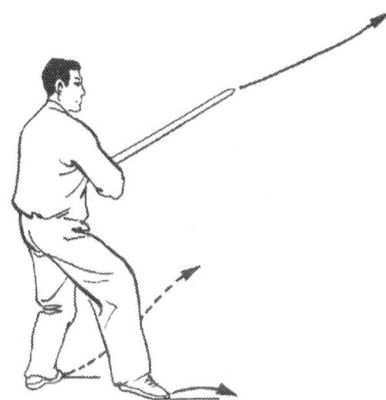

18

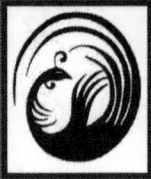

Form 8. Upward Pierce Sword with One-leg Stand

(19) Step your right foot forward, then stand on the right foot while lifting up the left leg, and move the sword upward in an independent stance. Fact east now (Figure 19).

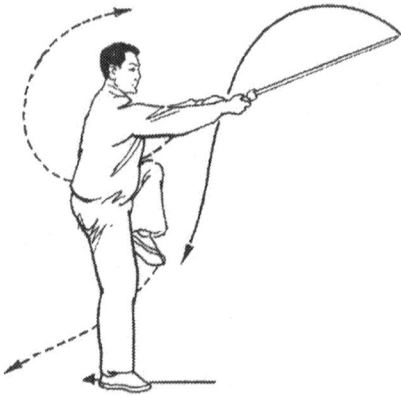

19

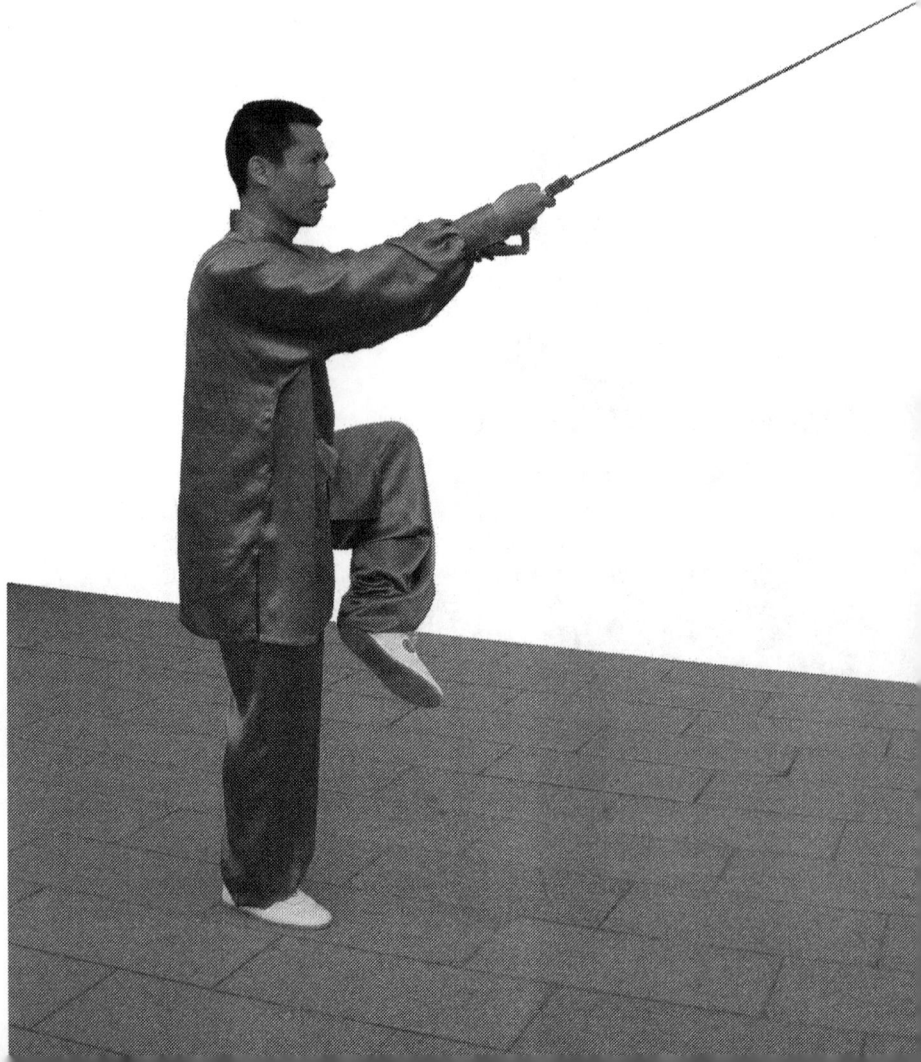

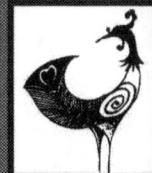

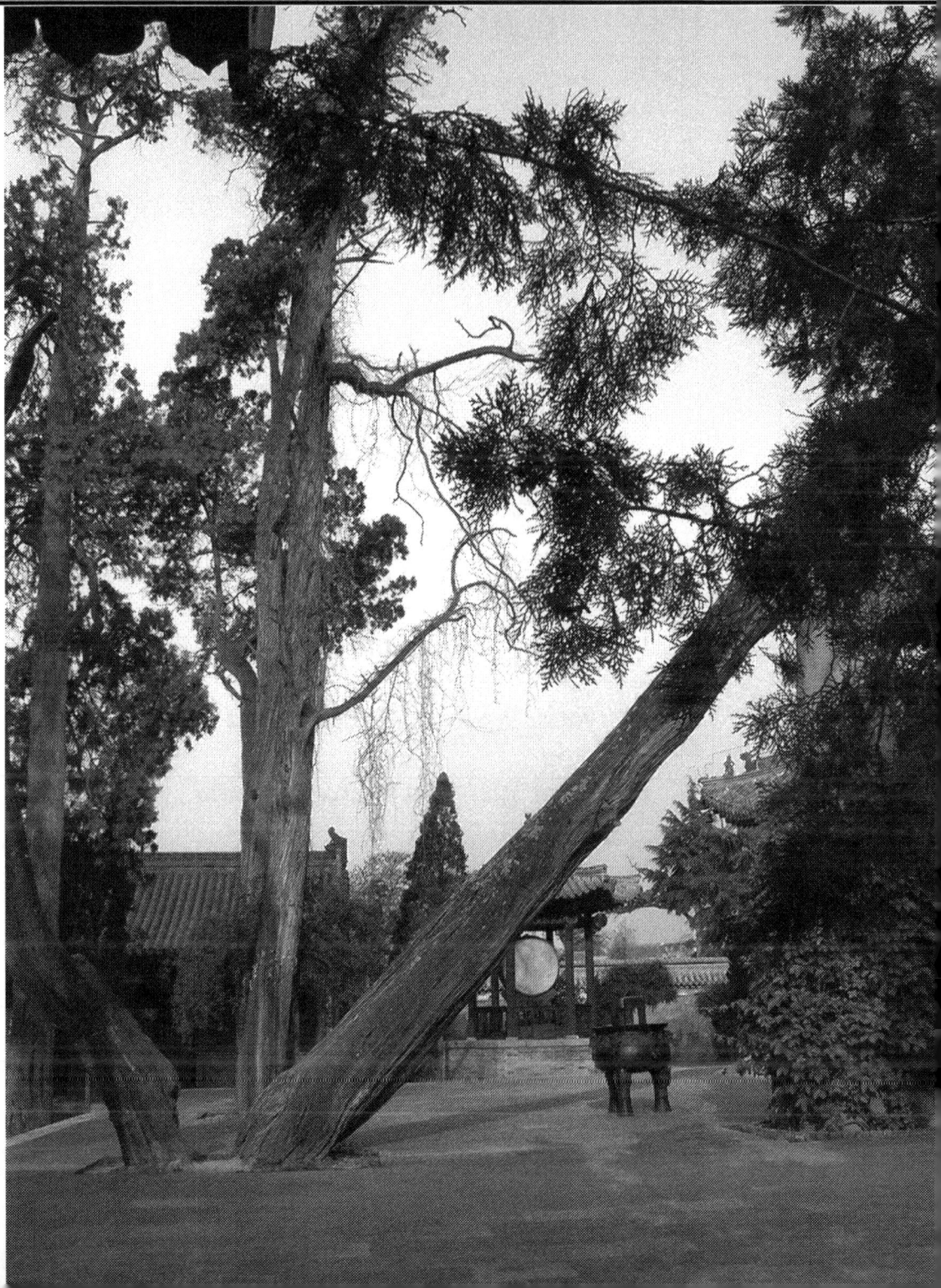

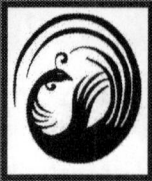

Group Two

The second group consists of eight forms shown below.

9.	Empty Stance and Slice Downward
10.	Pierce with Left Bow Stance
11.	Pull-back Turn and Skew Slice Sword
12.	Contract Body and Skew Slice Sword
13.	Raise Knee and Hold Sword
14.	Jump and Flat Pierce Forward
15.	Swing Sword with Left Empty Bow Stance
16.	Swing Sword with Right Bow Stance

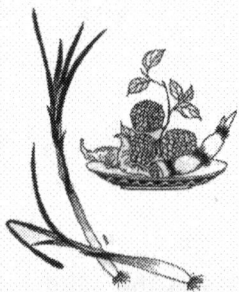

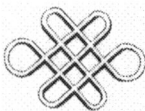

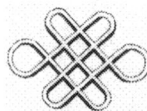

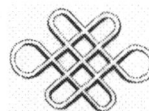

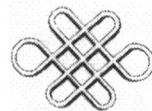

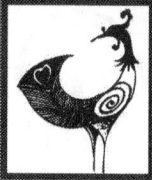

Form 9. Empty Stance and Slice Downward

(20) Step the left foot back to the left side and sit on the left leg in an empty stance while pulling both arms down, then the right hand cuts the sword downward and the left arm and hand circles upward. Face northeast (Figure 20).

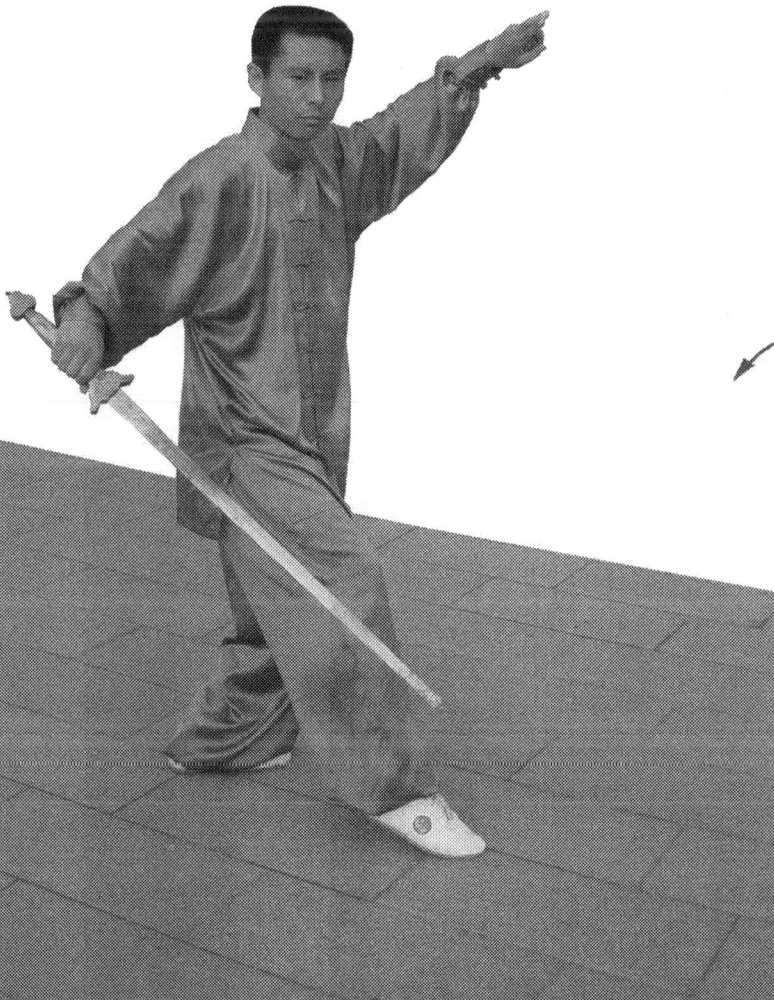

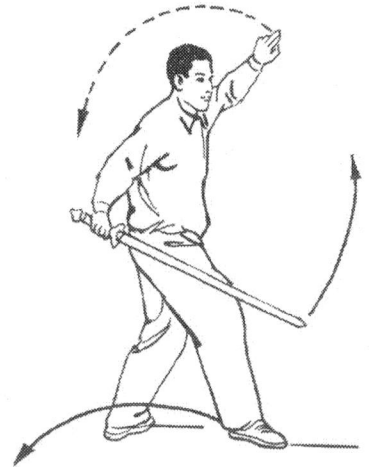

20

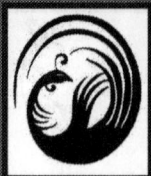

Form 10. Pierce with Left Bow Stance

(21) Step your right foot to the southwest side and then change your center to the right leg while drawing the sword to the right side. Direction: northeast (Figure 21).

(22) Lift the left leg, then step out on your left foot in a left bow stance to the northeast side and pierce the sword with the left arm upward. Face northeast (Figure 22).

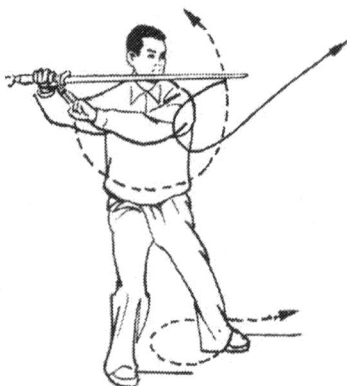

21

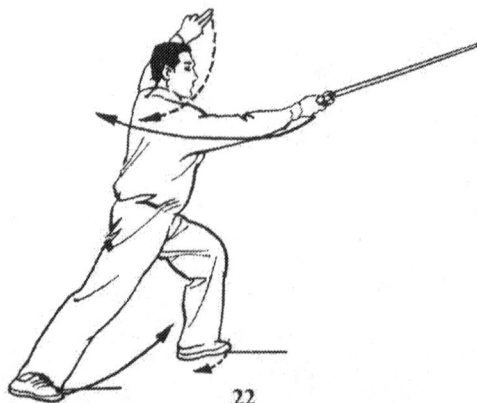

22

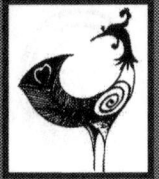

Figure 21. Step your right foot to the southwest side and then change your center to the right leg while drawing the sword to the right side. Face northeast.

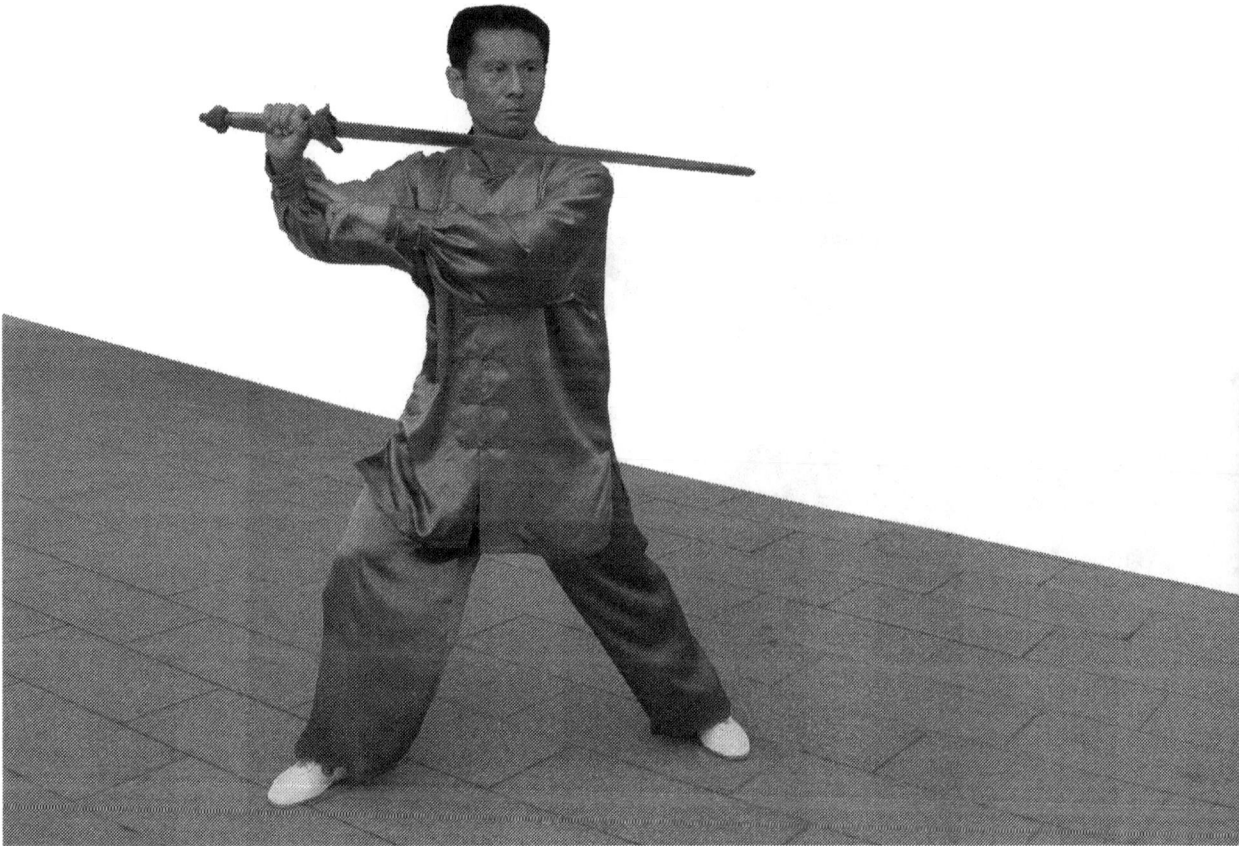

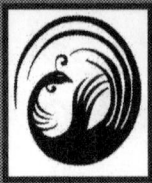

Figure 22. Lift the left leg, then step out on your left foot in a left bow stance to the northeast side and pierce the sword with the left arm upward. Face northeast.

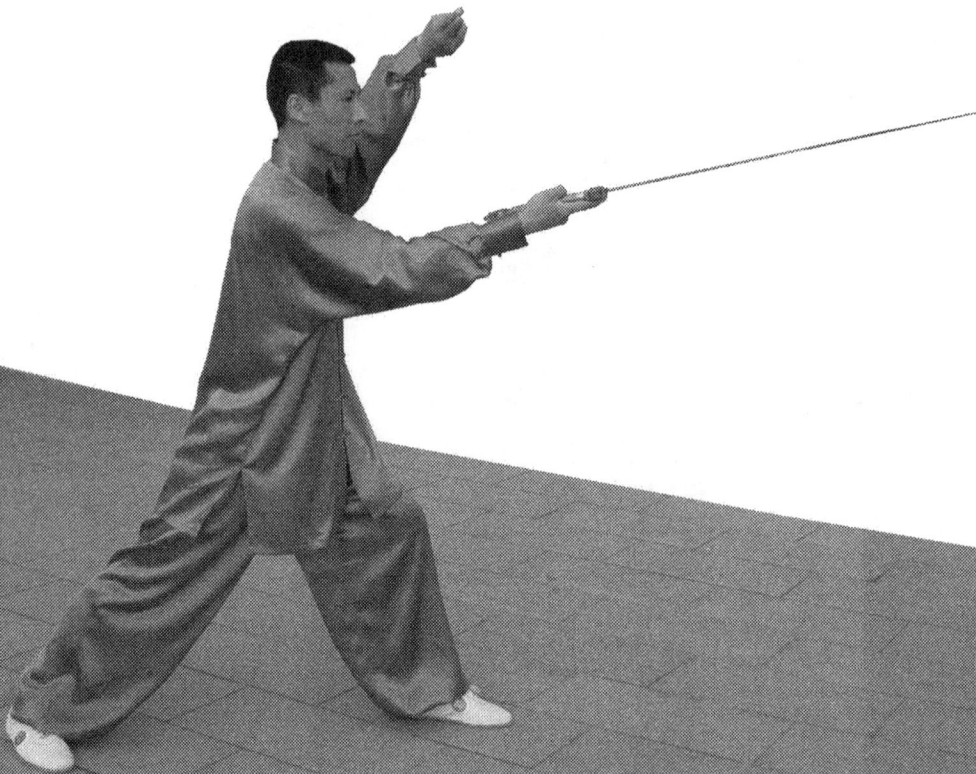

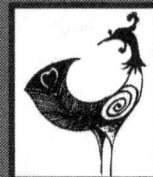

Form 11. Pull-back Turn and Skew Slice Sword

(23) Rotate your center (about 90 degrees) to your right side and stand on the left leg with the right leg lifting up. Face Southeast (Figure 23).

(24) Step out on your right foot with rotation (about 180 degrees) while circling and slicing the sword horizontally. Face northwest (Figure 24).

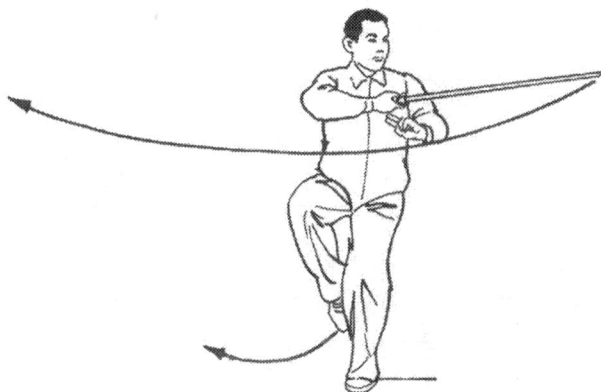

23

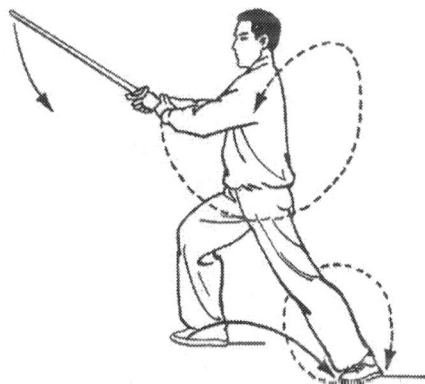

24

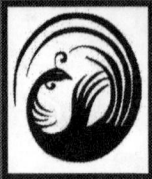

Figure 23. Rotate your center (about 90 degree) to right side and stand on the left leg with the right leg lifting up. Face southeast.

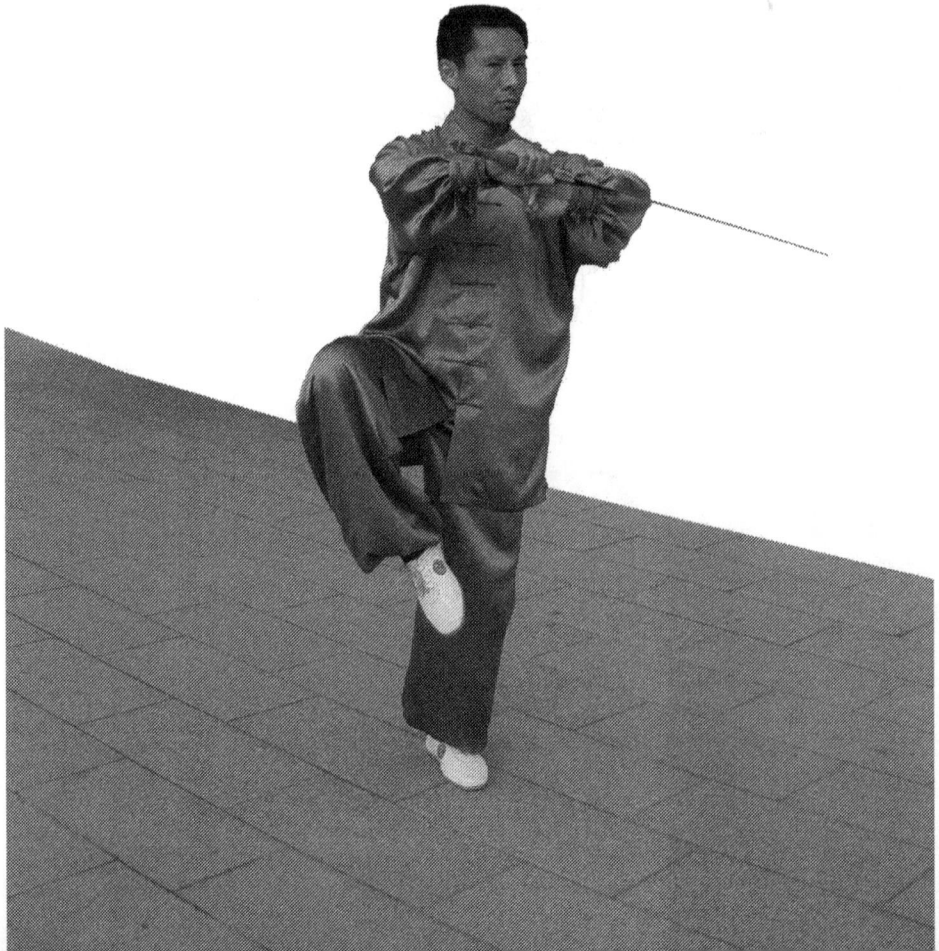

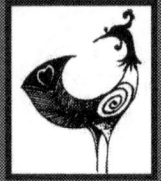

Figure 24. Step out with your right foot with rotation (about 180 degrees) while circling and slicing the sword horizontally. Face northwest.

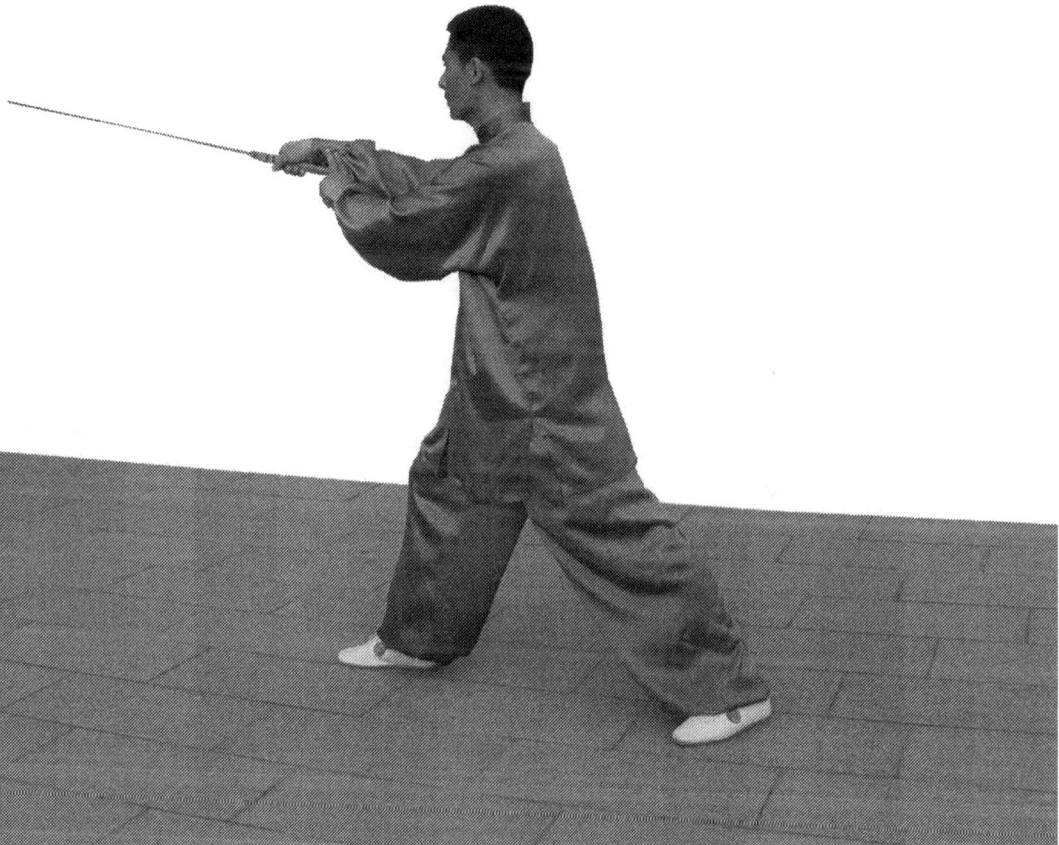

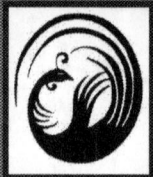
Form 12. Contract Body and Skew Slice Sword

(25) Shift your center back to the left leg while drawing the right foot beside the left foot, pulling the sword and circling the left hand in front of your chest. Face west (Figure 25). (26) Step your right foot backward and then sit on the right leg in an empty stance while slicing the sword backward with separation of both arms. Face west (Figure 26).

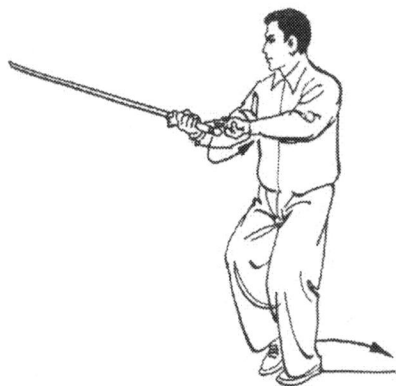

25

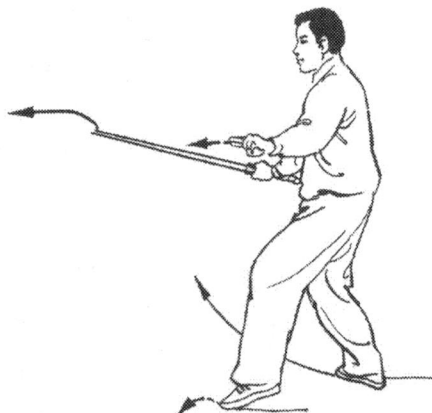

26

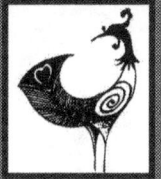

Figure 25. Shift your center back to the left leg while drawing the right foot beside the left foot, pulling the sword and circling the left hand in front of your chest. Face west.

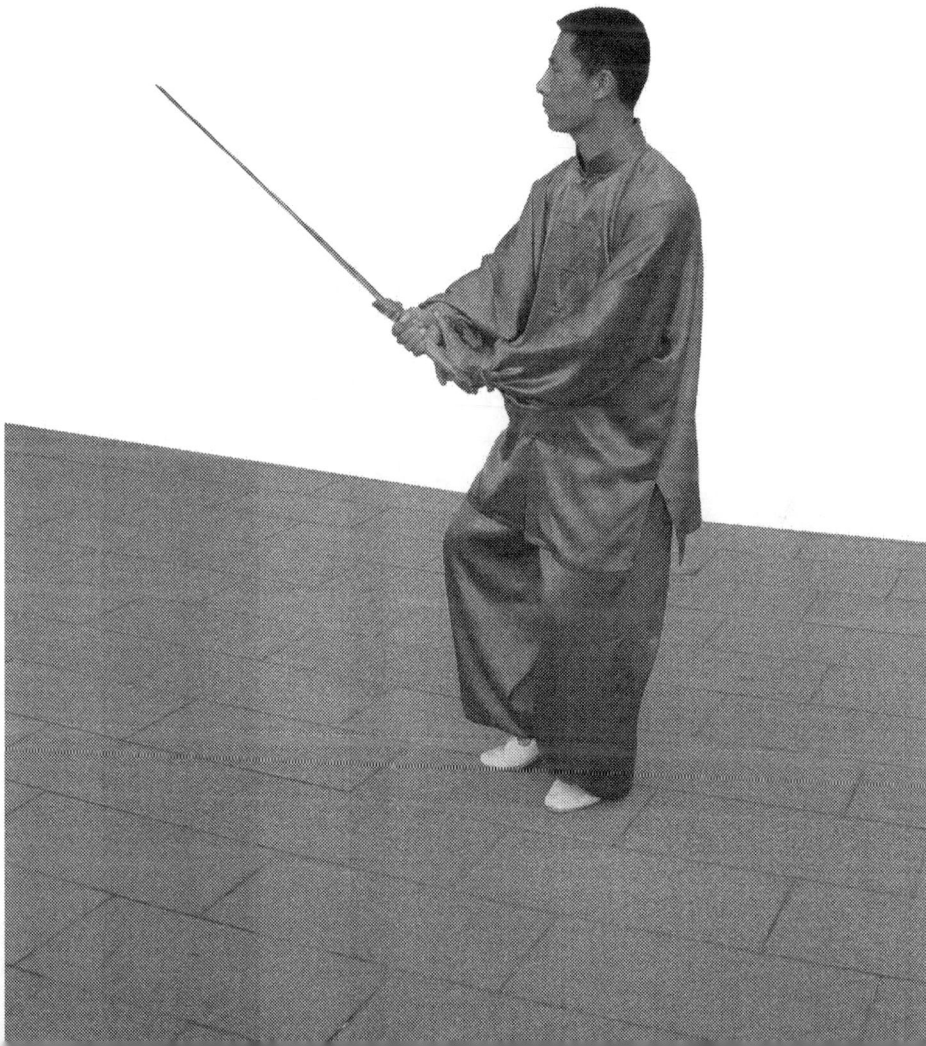

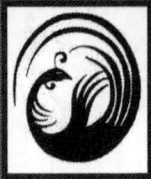

Figure 26. Step your right foot backward and then sit on the right leg in an empty stance while slicing the sword backward with separation of both arms. Face west.

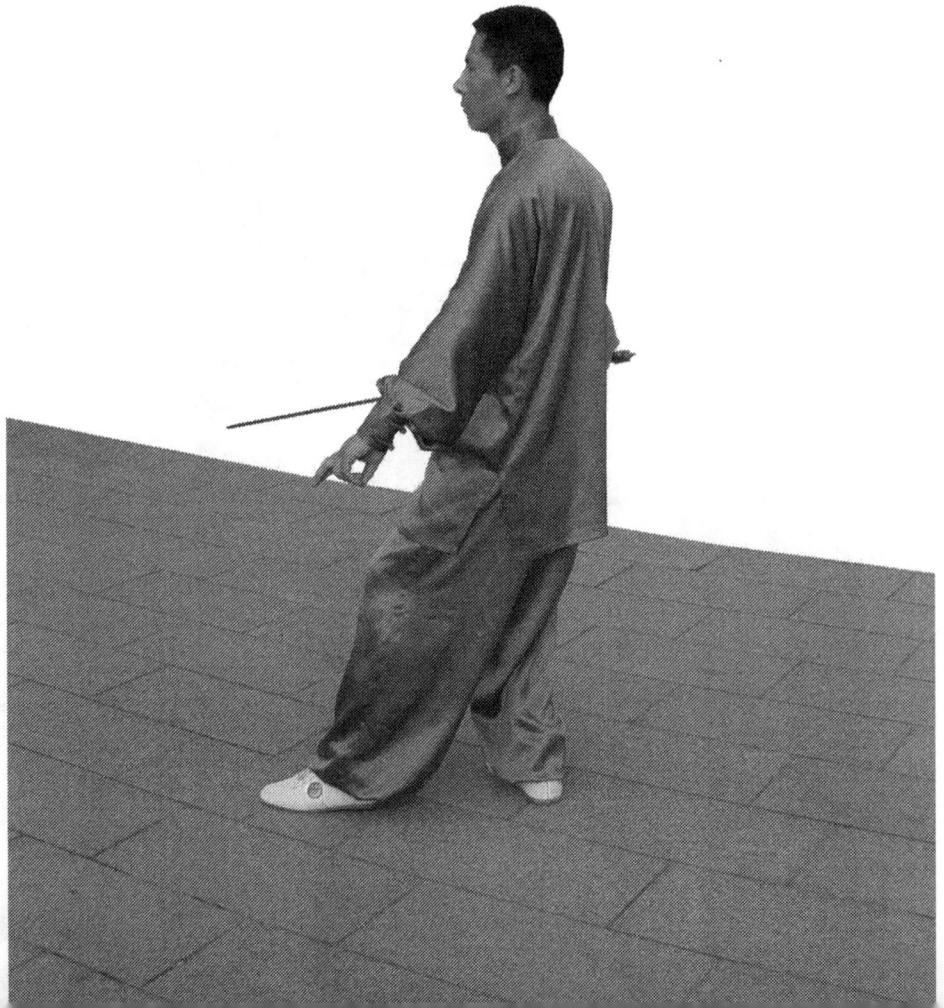

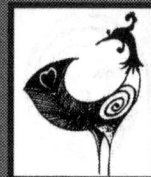

Form 13. Raise Knee and Hold Sword

(27) Step forward with the left foot and then stand on the left leg while holding the sword in front of your chest. Face west (Figure 27).

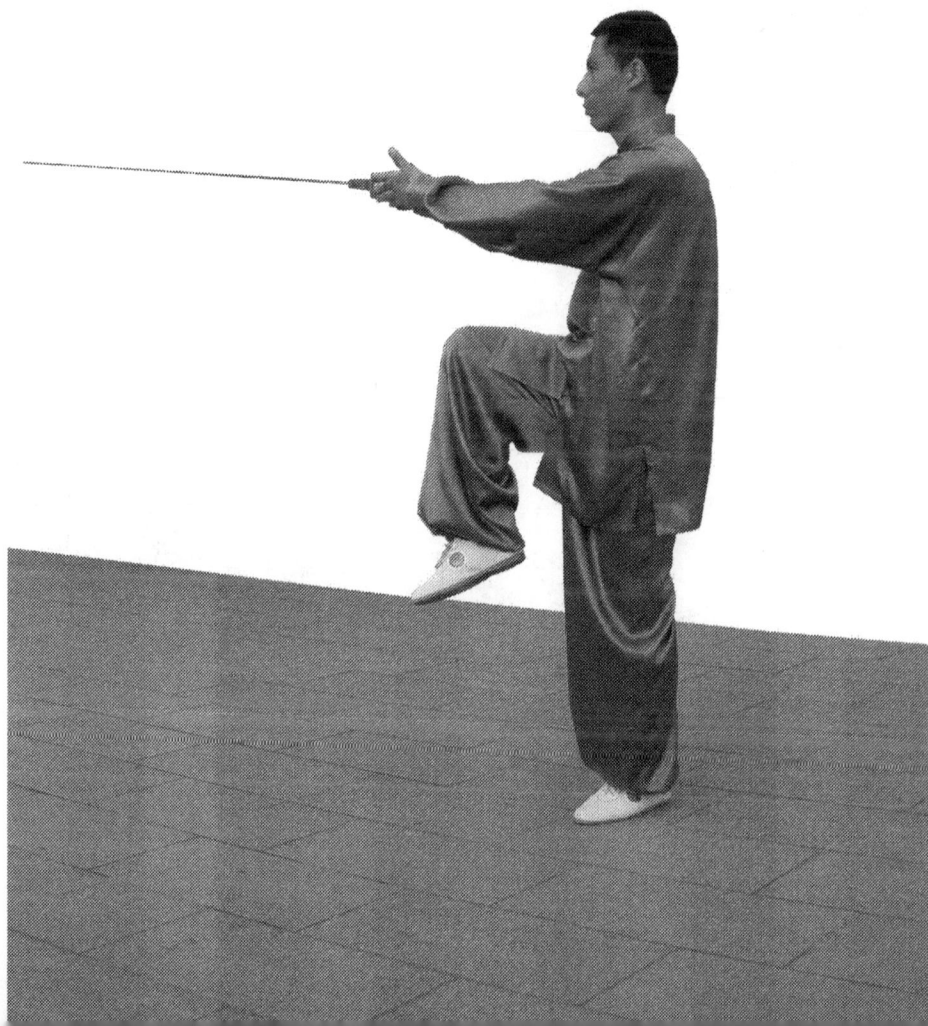

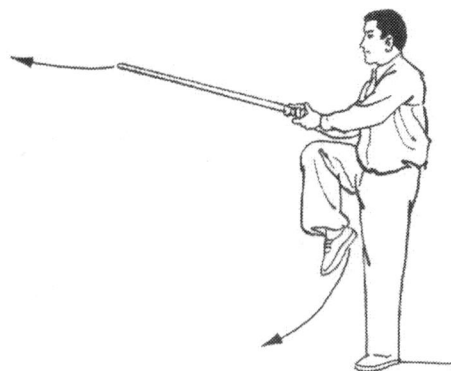

27

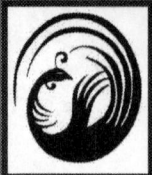

Form 14. Jump and Flat Pierce Forward

(28) Put down the right foot and stand on the right foot while sending the sword forward. Face west (Figure 28).

(29) Jump with the left foot while pulling down both arms and lifting the right foot. Face west (Figure 29).

(30) Step your right foot forward in a right bow stance while piercing the sword forward flatly. Face west (Figure 30).

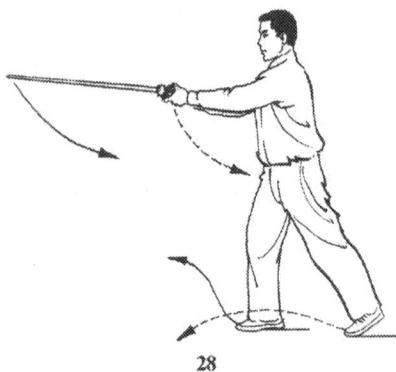

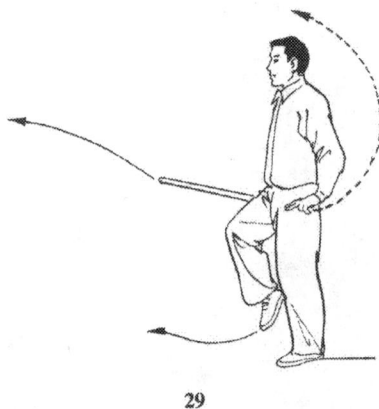

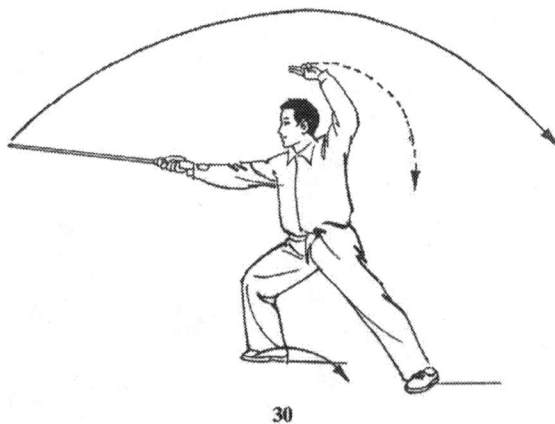

28

29

30

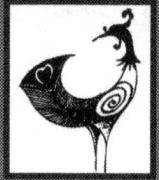

Figure 28. Put down the right foot and stand on the right foot while sending the sword forward. Face west.

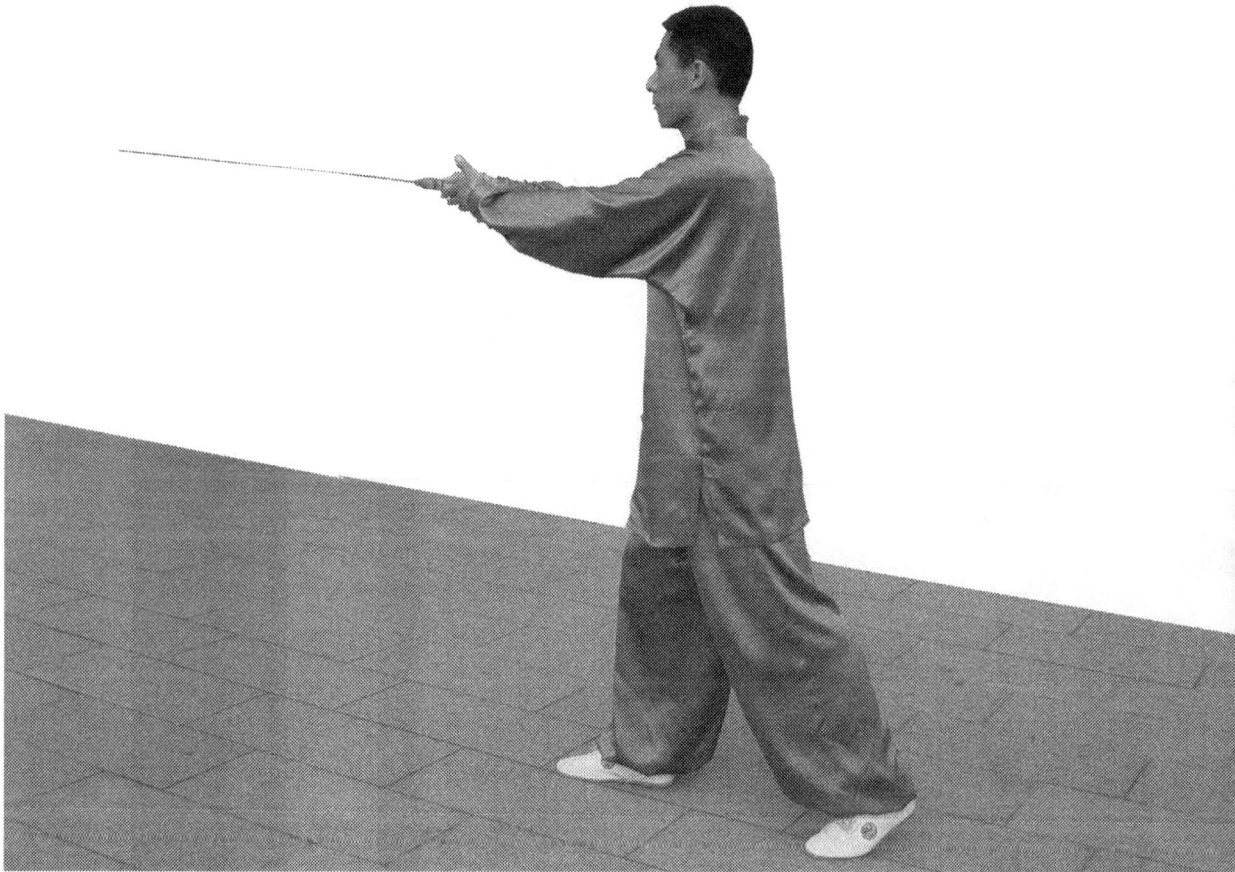

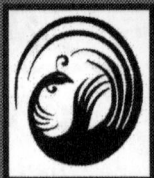

Figure 29. Jump with the left foot while pulling down both arms and lifting the right foot. Face west.

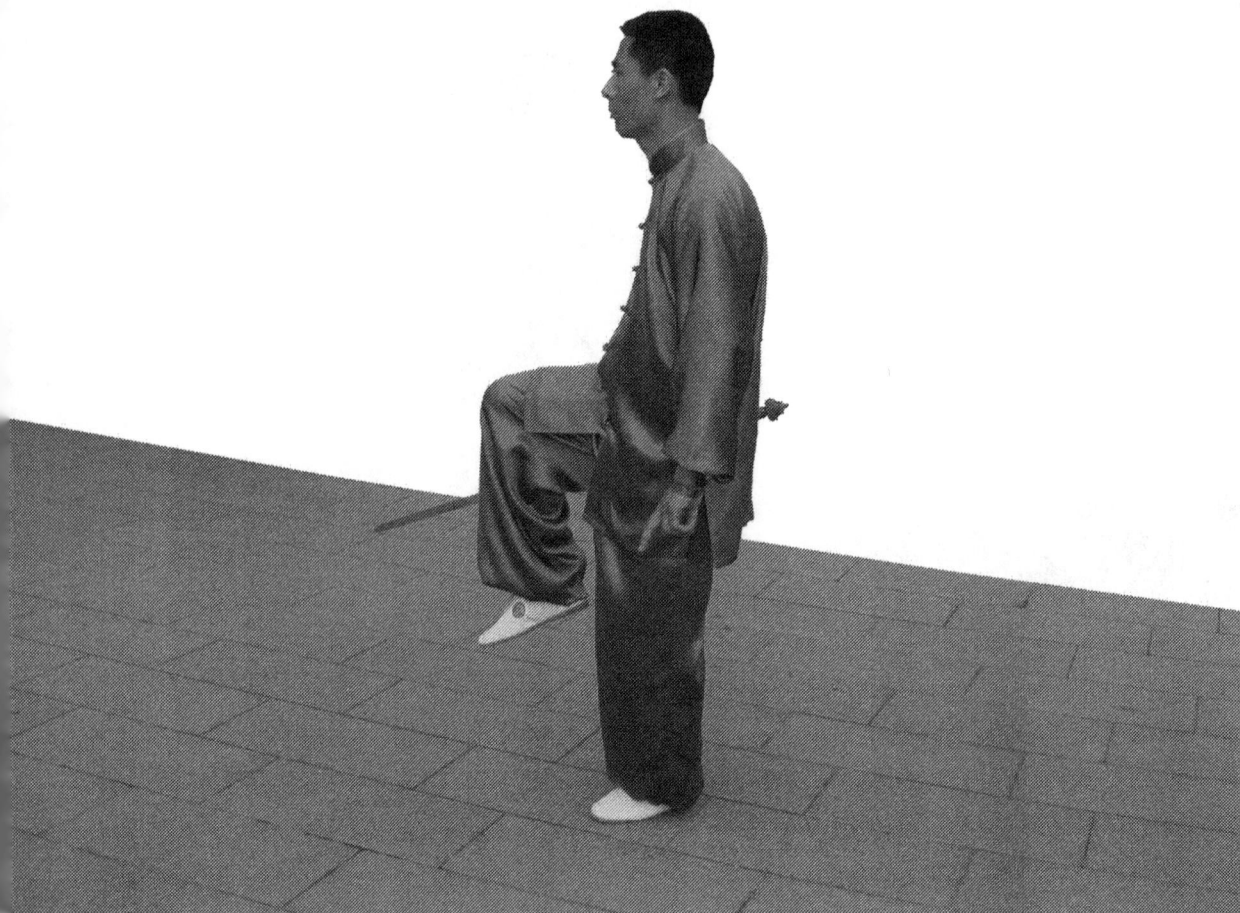

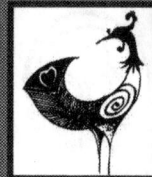

Figure 30. Step your right foot forward in a right bow stance while piercing the sword forward flatly. Face west.

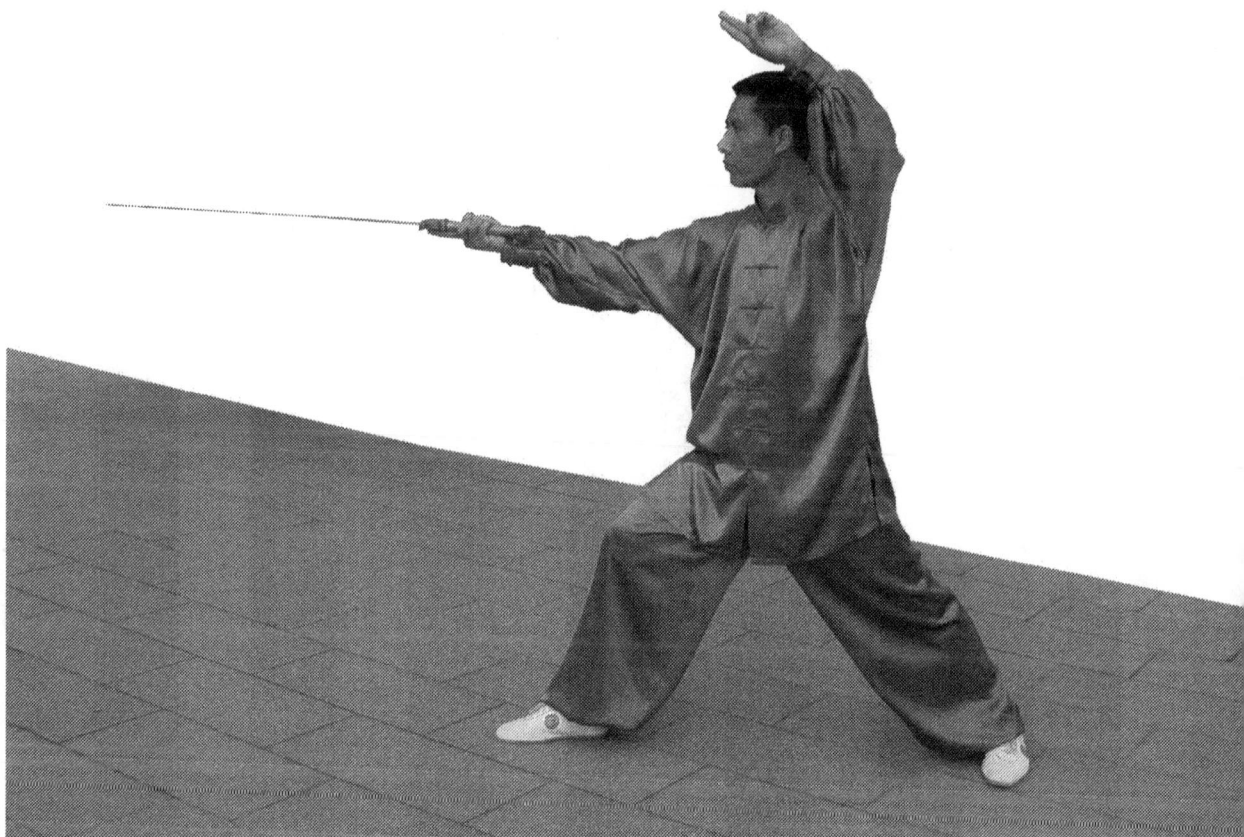

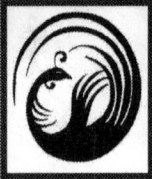
Form 15. Swing Sword with Left Empty Bow Stance

(31) Shift the center to the left leg while drawing back the right foot close to the left foot and circling the sword and left hand to the left side of your waist. Face southeast (Figure 31).

(32) Step out with the right foot and transfer the center to the right leg in a sit-on stance while sending the left foot forward in a right empty stance. Face west (Figure 32).

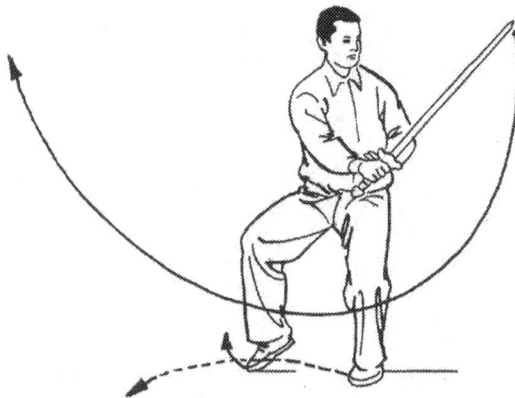

31

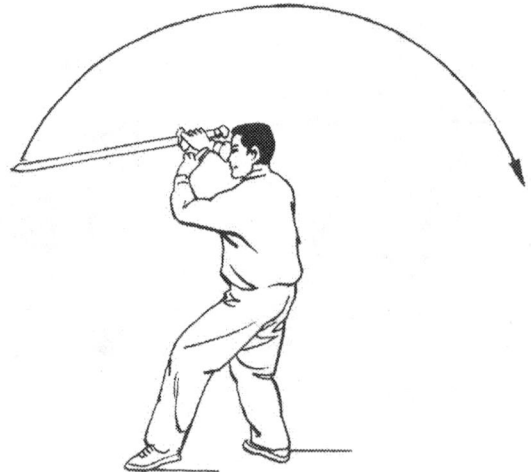

32

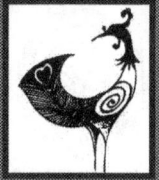

Figure 31. Shift the center to the left leg while drawing back the right foot close to the left foot and circling the sword and left hand to the left side of your waist. Face southeast.

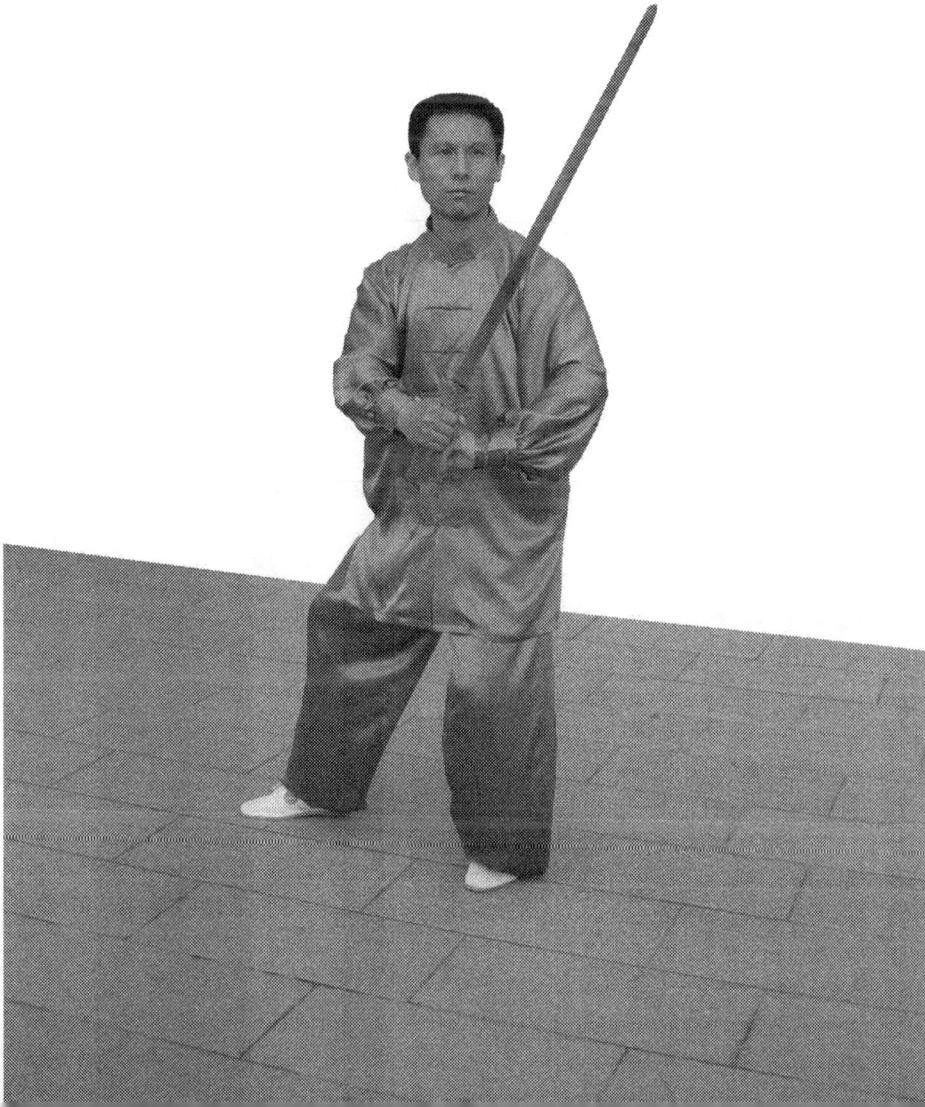

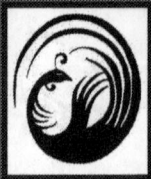

Figure 32.   Step out the right foot and transfer the center to the right leg in a sit-on stance while sending the left foot forward in a right empty stance. Face west.

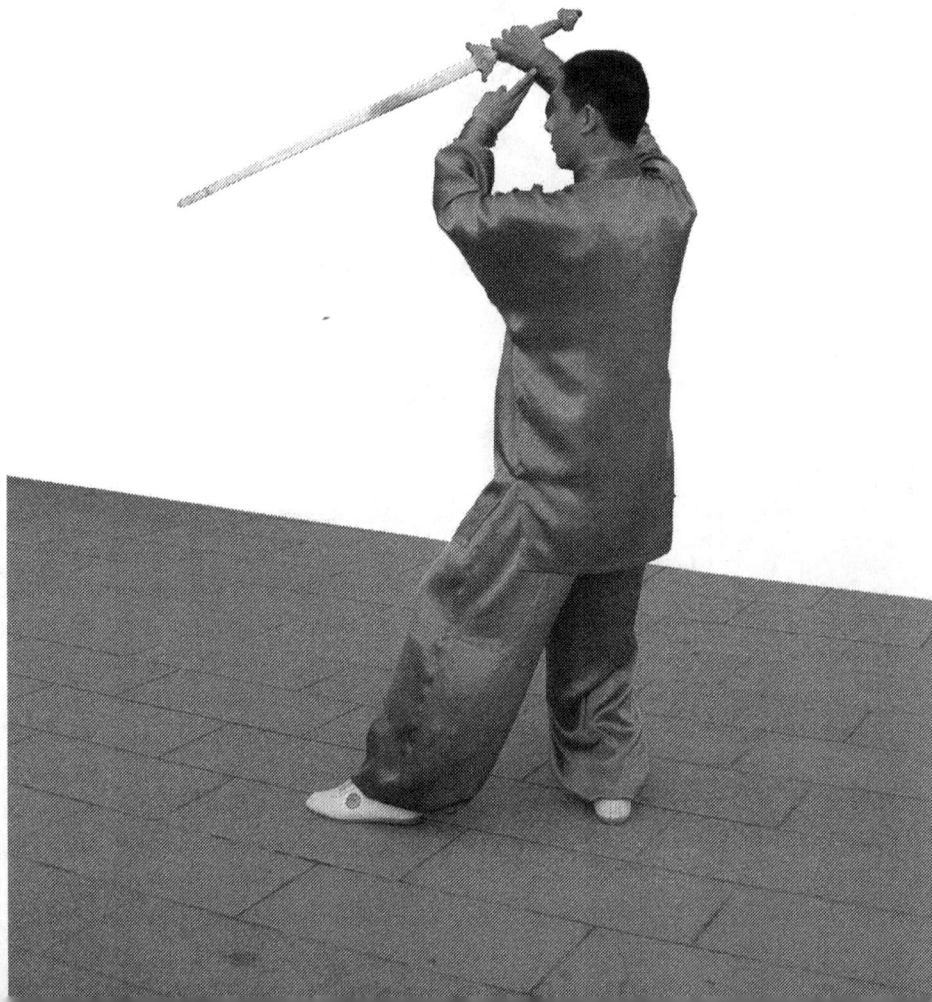

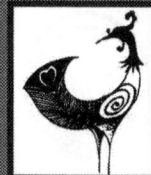

Form 16. Swing Sword with Right Bow Stance

(33) Circle the sword backward to the northeast direction while keeping the left empty stance (Figure 33).

(34) Step out the left foot a little, then shift center to the left leg and move the right foot forward to form the right bow stance while swinging the sword and circling the left arm upward. Face west (Figure 34).

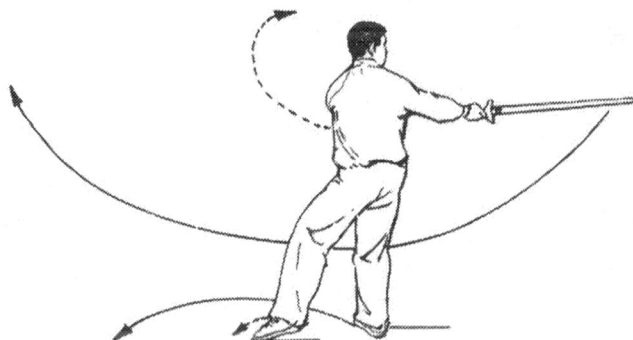

33

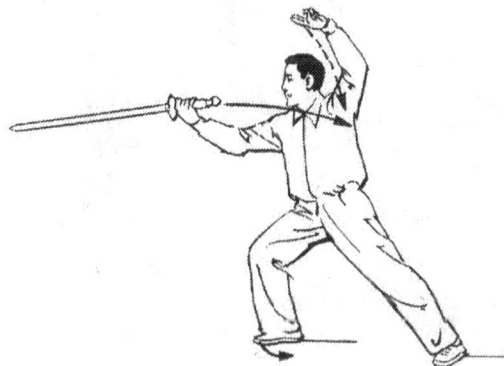

34

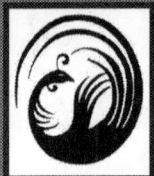

Figure 33. Circle the sword backward to the northeast direction while keeping the left empty stance.

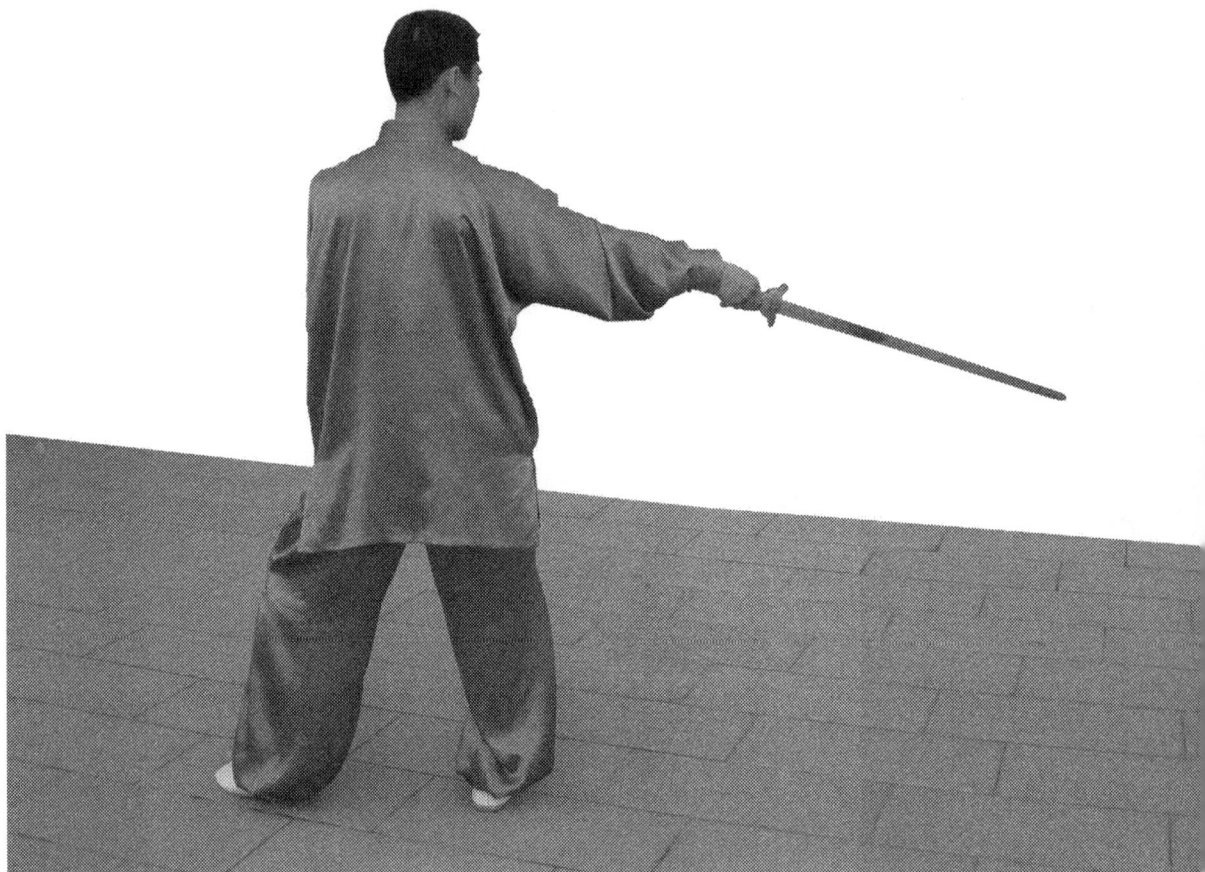

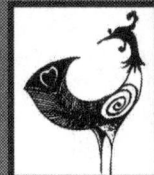

Figure 34. Step out the left foot a little, then shift center to the left leg and move the right foot forward to form the right bow stance while swinging the sword and circling the left arm upward. Face west.

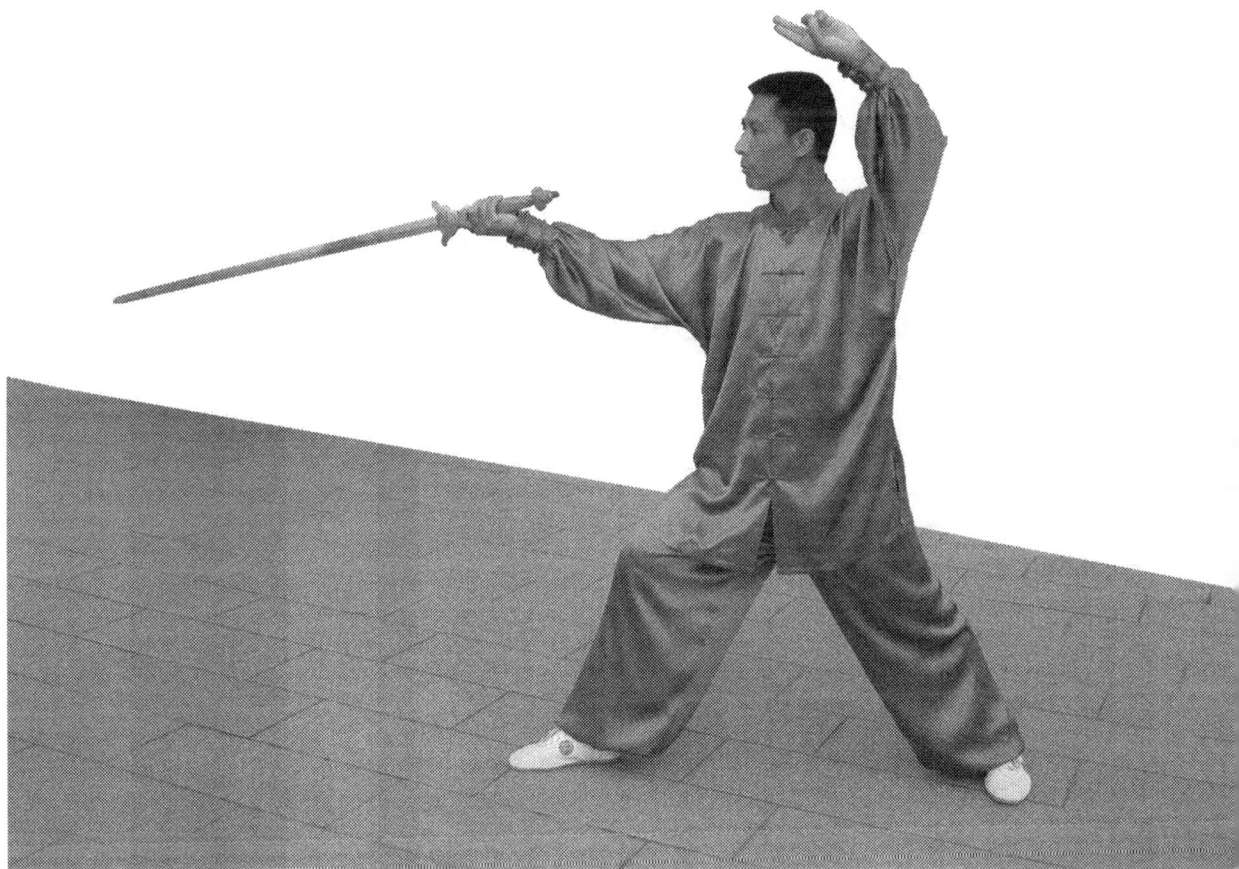

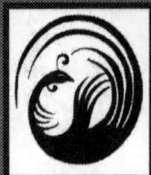

Group Three

The third group consists of eight forms shown below.

17. *Turn and Pull Sword Back*
18. *Close Steps and Flat Pierce*
19. *Obstruct Sword with Left Bow Stance*
20. *Obstruct Sword with Right Bow Stance*
21. *Obstruct Sword with Left Bow Stance*
22. *Step Forward and Opposite Pierce*
23. *Reposition and Chop Back*
24. *Point Sword with Empty Stance*

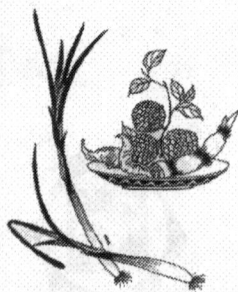

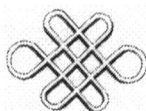

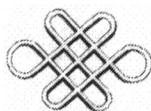

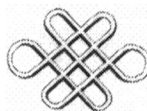

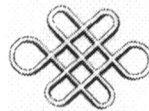

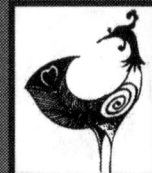

Form 17. Turn and Pull Sword Back

(35) Shift your center to your left leg and rotate your body to your left side with the left hand beside the right hand while circling the sword to the southeast direction (Figure 35).
(36) Chop the sword in a left bow stance. Face southeast (Figure 36).

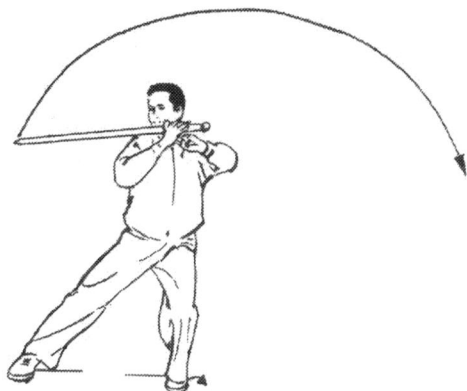

(37) Shift back to the right leg in a left empty stance while pulling the sword backward and pointing the left hand fingers out. Face south-east (Figure 37).

35

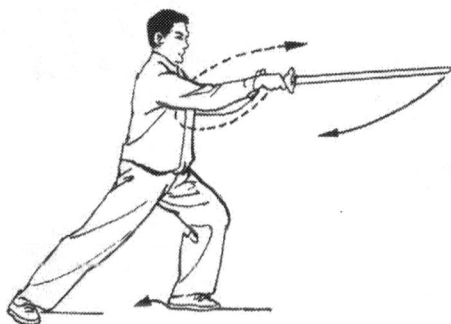

36

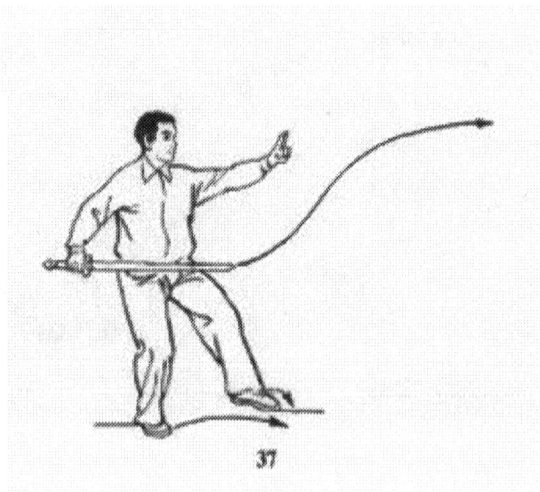

37

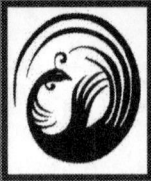

Figure 35. Shift your center to your left leg and rotate your body to your left side with the left hand beside the right hand while circling the sword to the southeast direction.

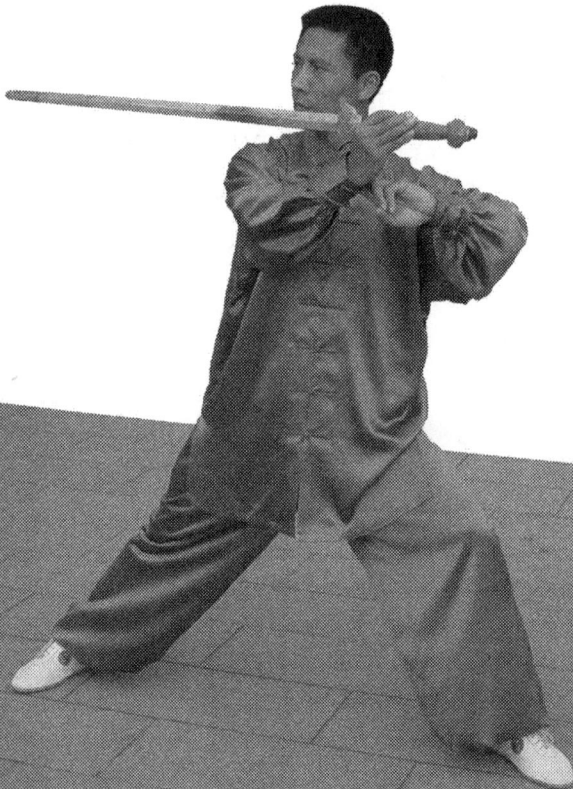

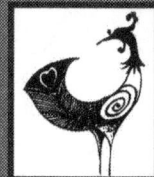

Figure 36. Chop the sword in a left bow stance. Face south-east.

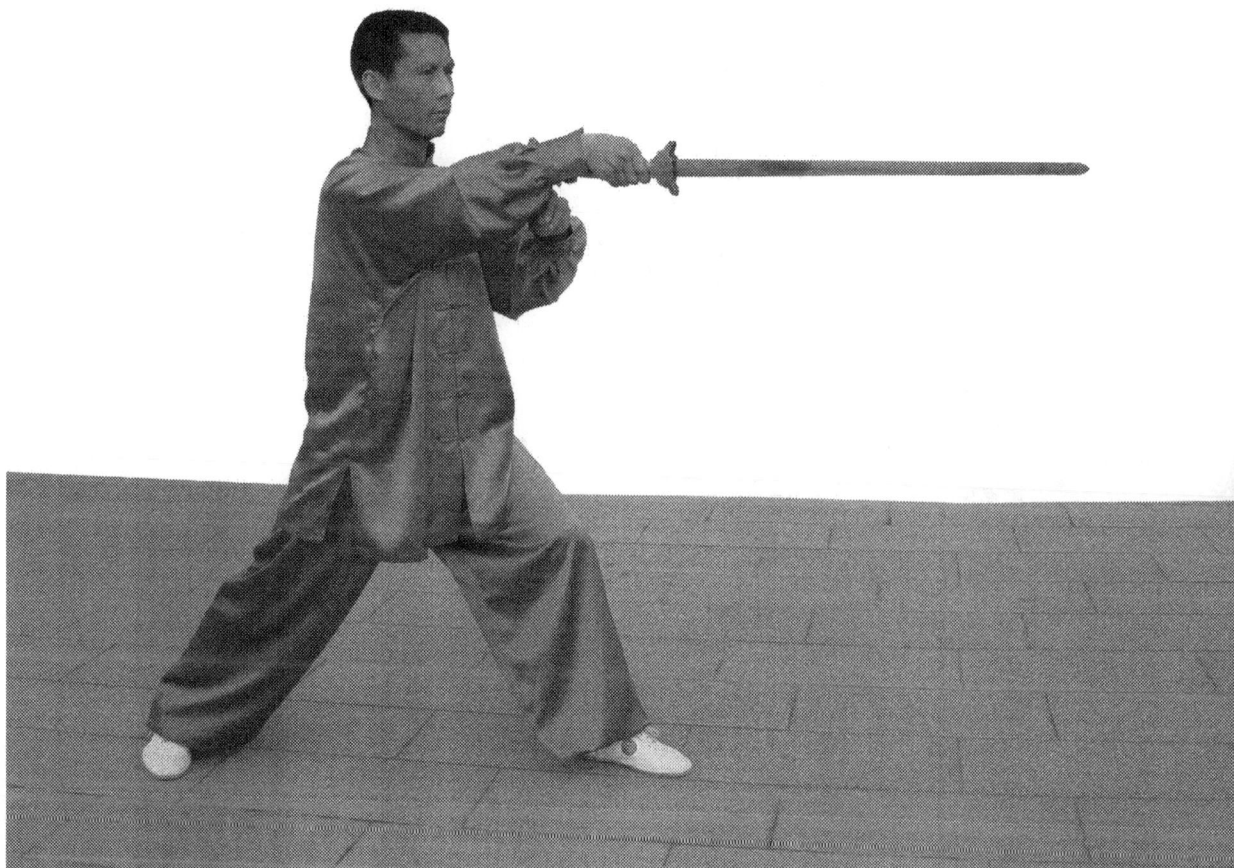

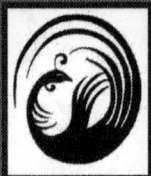

Figure 37. Shift back to the right leg in a left empty stance while pulling the sword backward and pointing the left hand fingers out. Face southeast.

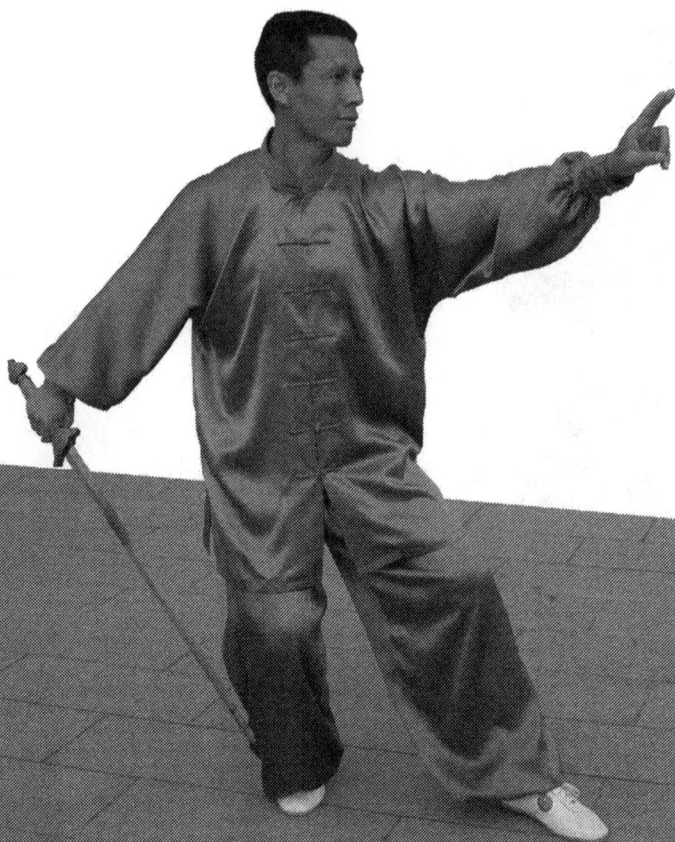

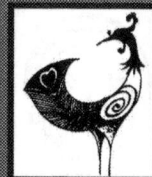

Form 18. Close Steps and Flat Pierce

(38) Step out on the left foot a little and then draw your right foot to the left foot while piercing the sword forward horizontally with both hands touching together. Face east (Figure 38).

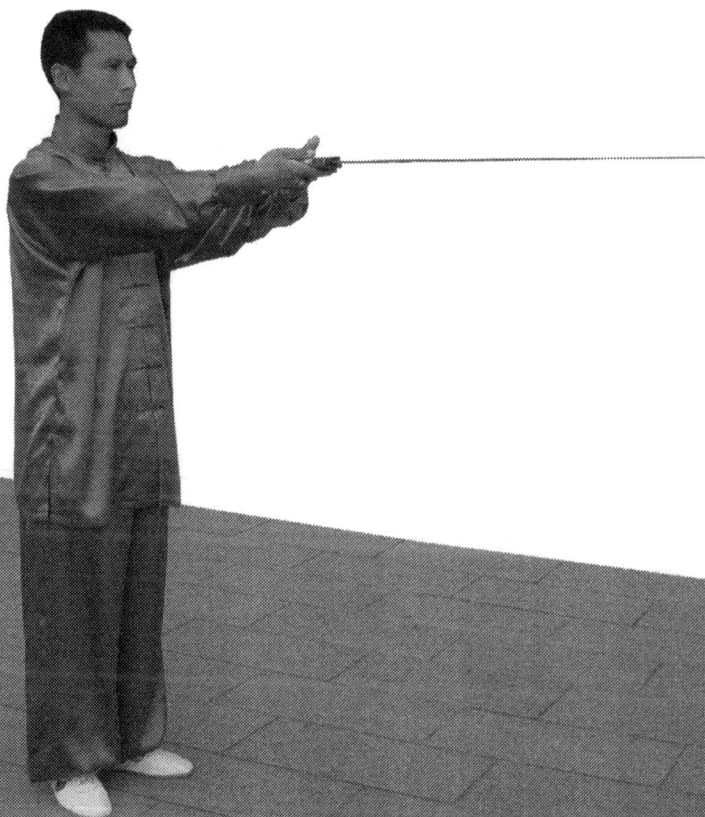

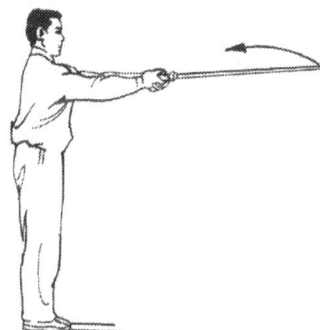

38

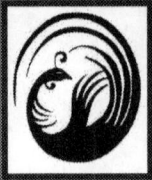

Form 19. Obstruct Sword with Left Bow Stance

(39) Step out with your left foot while circling the sword backward. Face southeast (Figure 39).

(40) Change to left bow stance and obstruct the sword while circling the left arm upward. Face east (Figure 40).

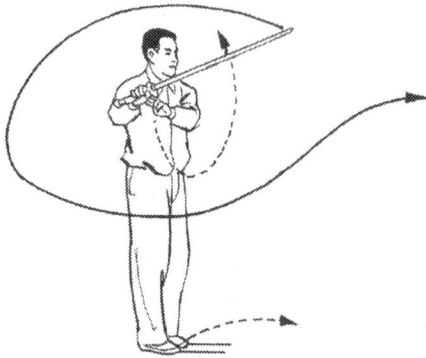

39

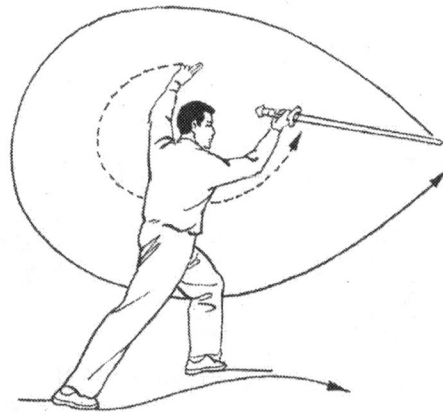

40

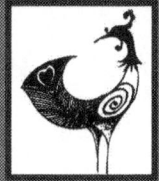

Figure 39. Step out on your left foot while circling the sword backward. Face southeast.

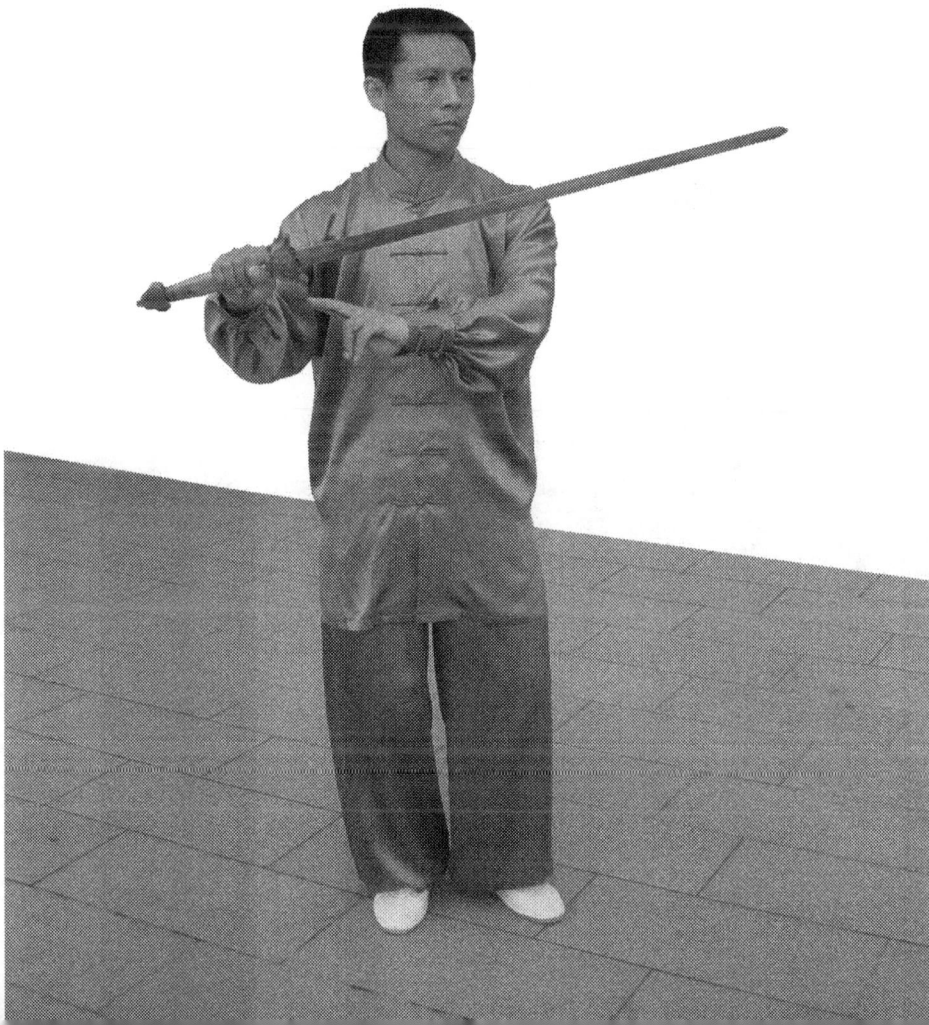

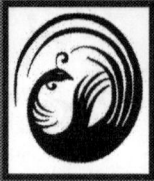

Figure 40. Change to left bow stance and obstruct the sword while circling the left arm upward. Face east.

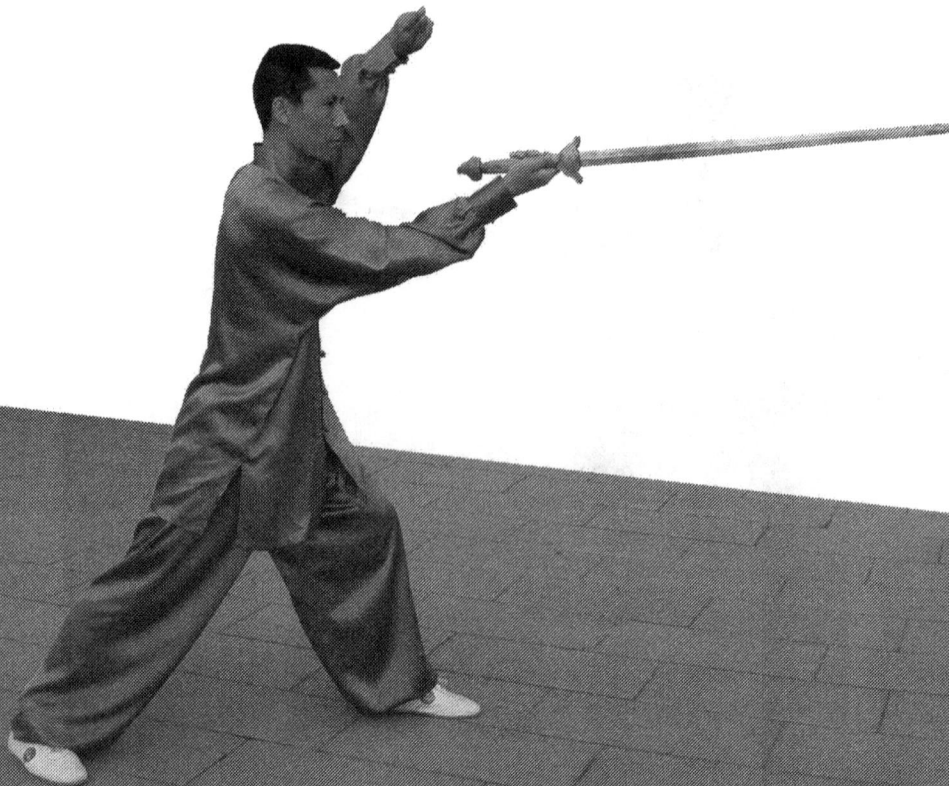

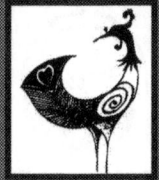

Form 20. Obstruct Sword with Right Bow Stance

(41) Step out with your right foot while circling the sword backward to the left side; Change to the right bow stance and obstruct the sword with the left hand touching the right hand. Face west (Figure 41).

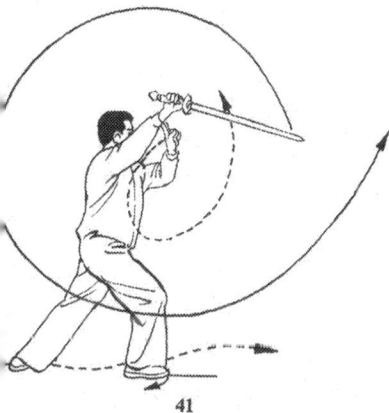

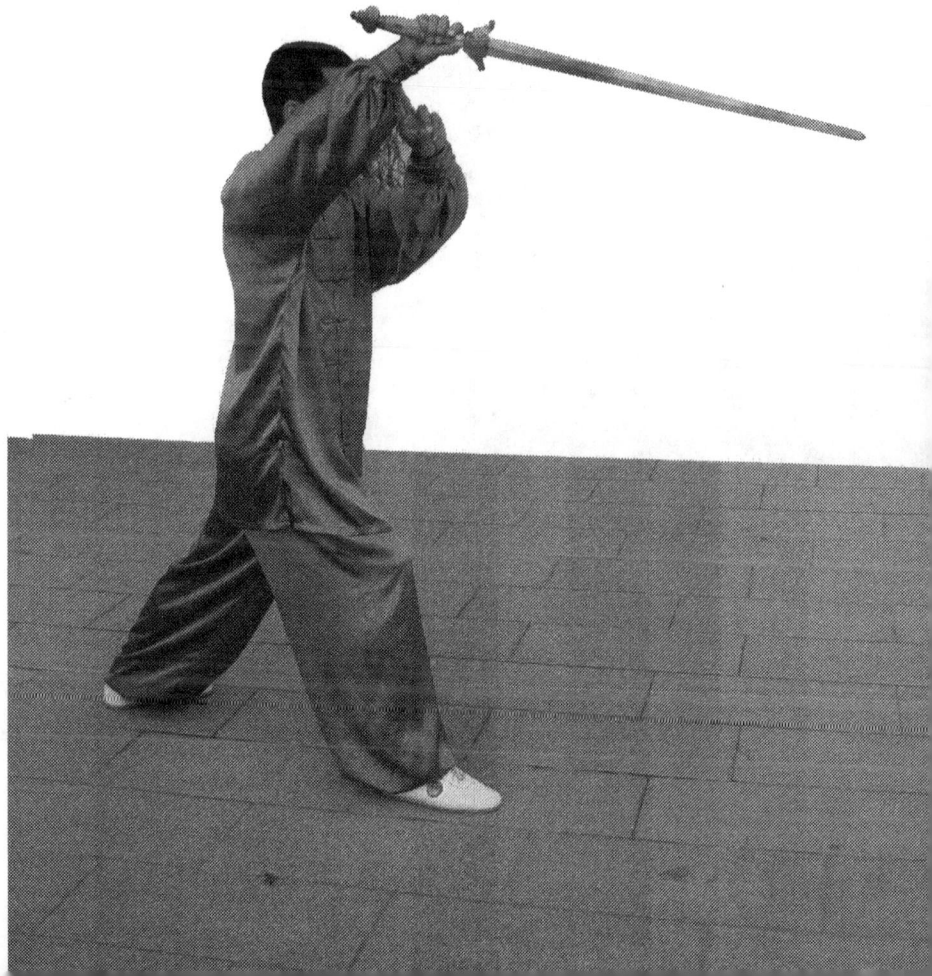

41

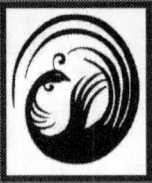

Form 21. Obstruct Sword with Left Bow Stance

(42) Step out your left foot while circling the sword backward; Change to the left bow stance and obstruct the sword forward with the left arm upward. Face west (Figure 42).

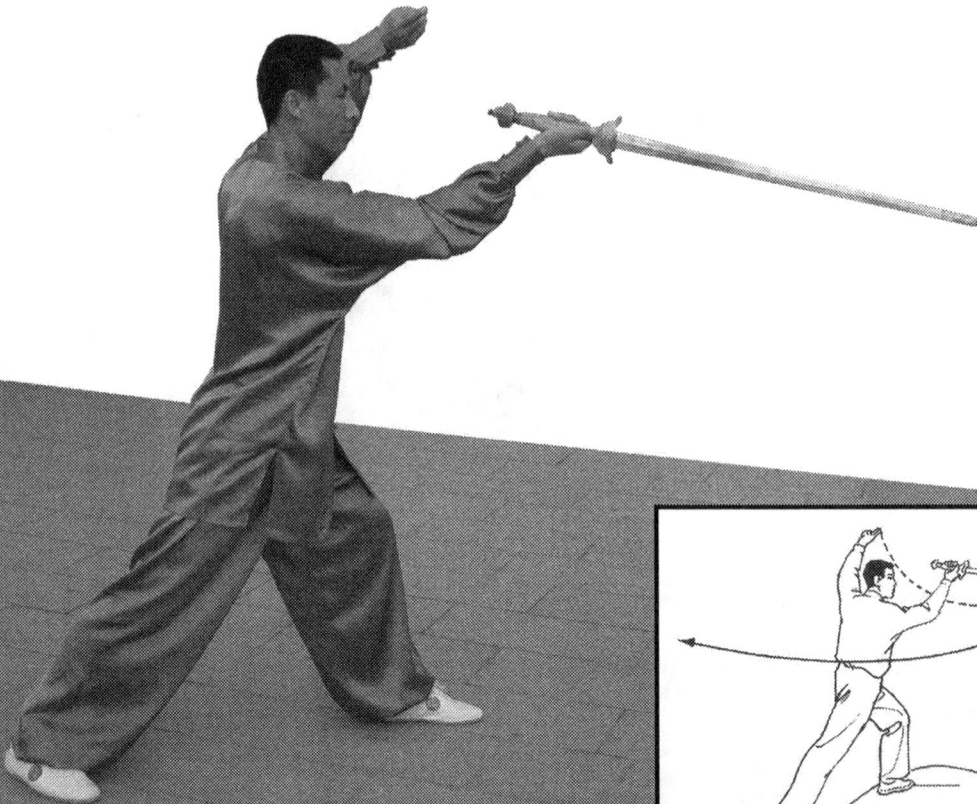

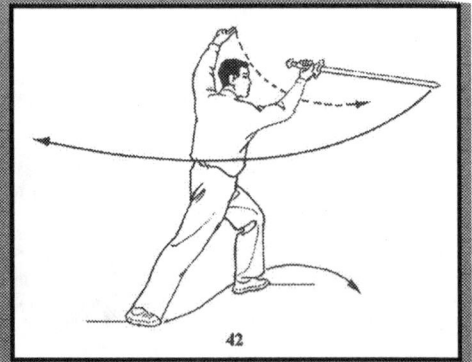

42

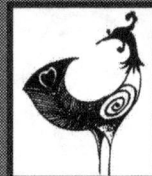

Form 22. Step Forward and Opposite Pierce

(43) Lift your right foot forward in a resting stance while extending the right arm backward and the left arm forward. Face west (Figure 43).

(44) Lift your left foot forward in a left bow stance while piercing the sword backward with both hands touching each other. Face east (Figure 44).

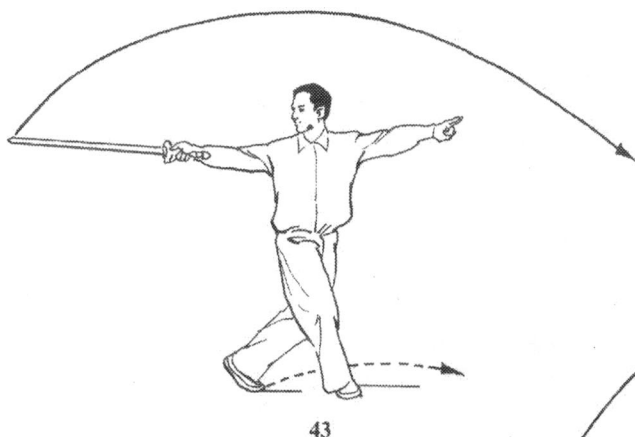

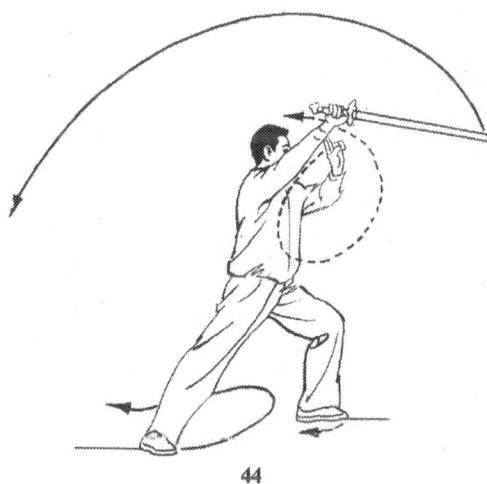

43

44

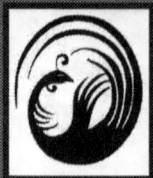

Figure 43. Lift your right foot forward in a resting stance while extending the right arm backward and the left arm forward. Face west.

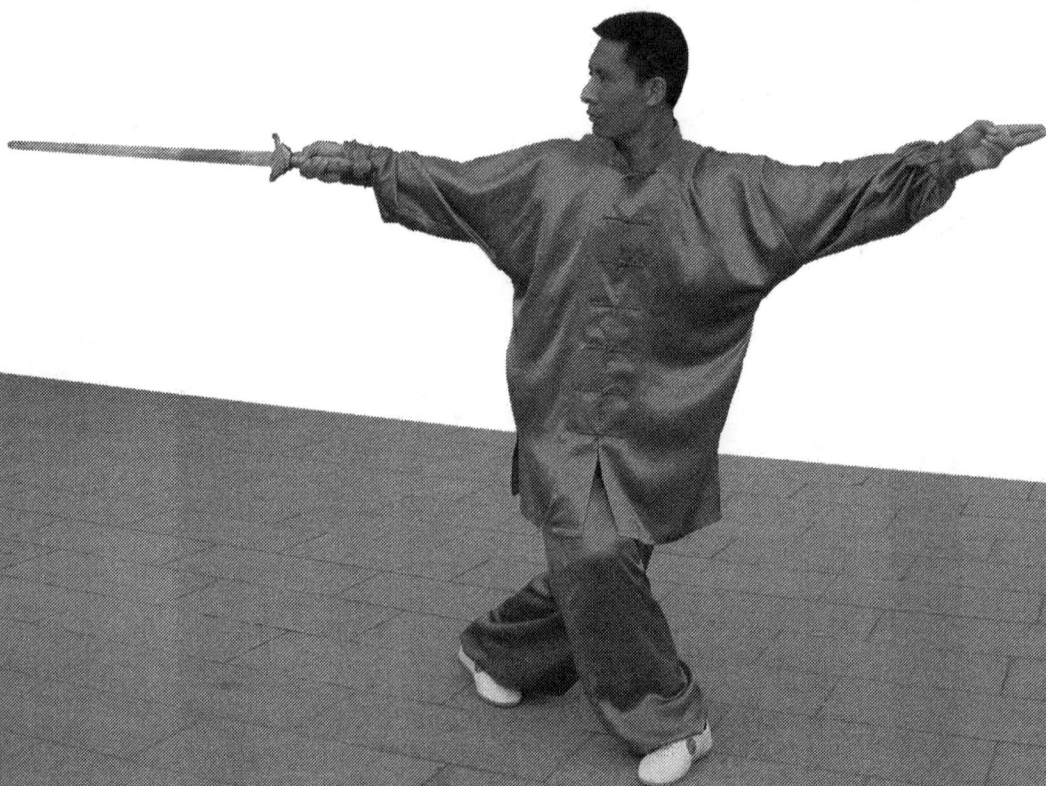

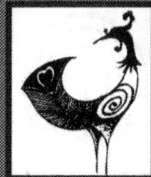

Figure 44. Lift your left foot forward in a left bow stance while piercing the sword backward with both hands touching each other. Face east.

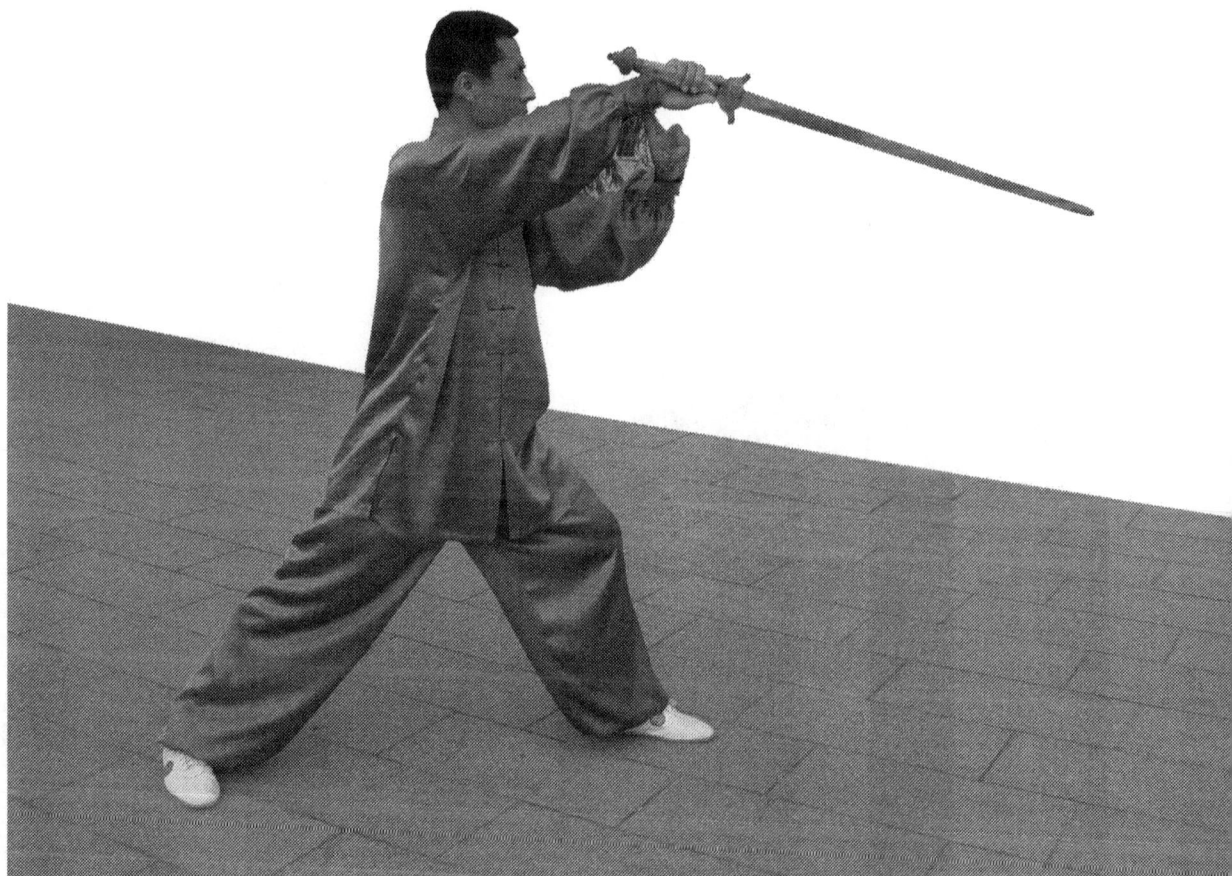

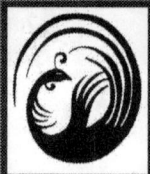

Form 23. Reposition and Chop Back

(45) Shift your center to the left leg and then shift the center back to the right leg while rotating your body to the right. Lift your right foot forward in a right bow stance while chopping the sword. Face northwest (Figure 45).

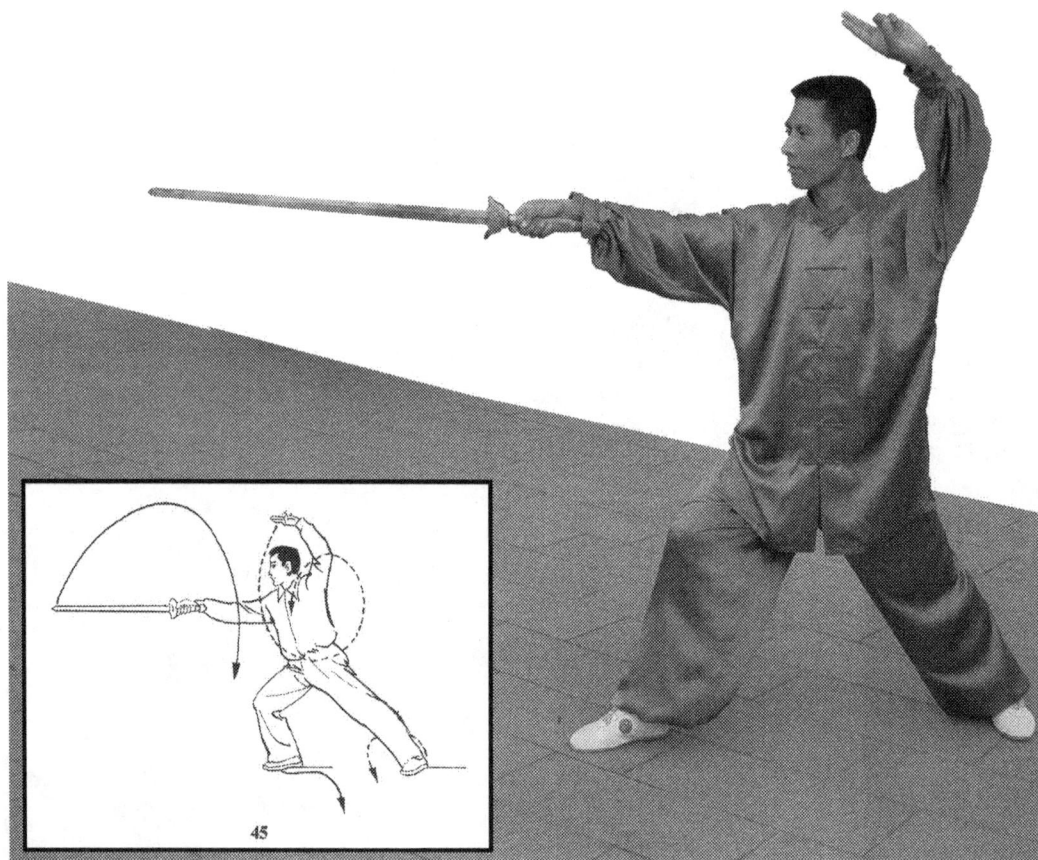

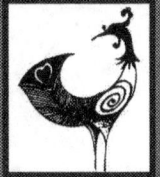

Form 24. Point Sword with Empty Stance

(46) Lift your left foot and place it on the south side, then sit on the left leg in a right empty stance with the right foot placed forward while circling both arms and pointing the sword. Face south (Figure 46).

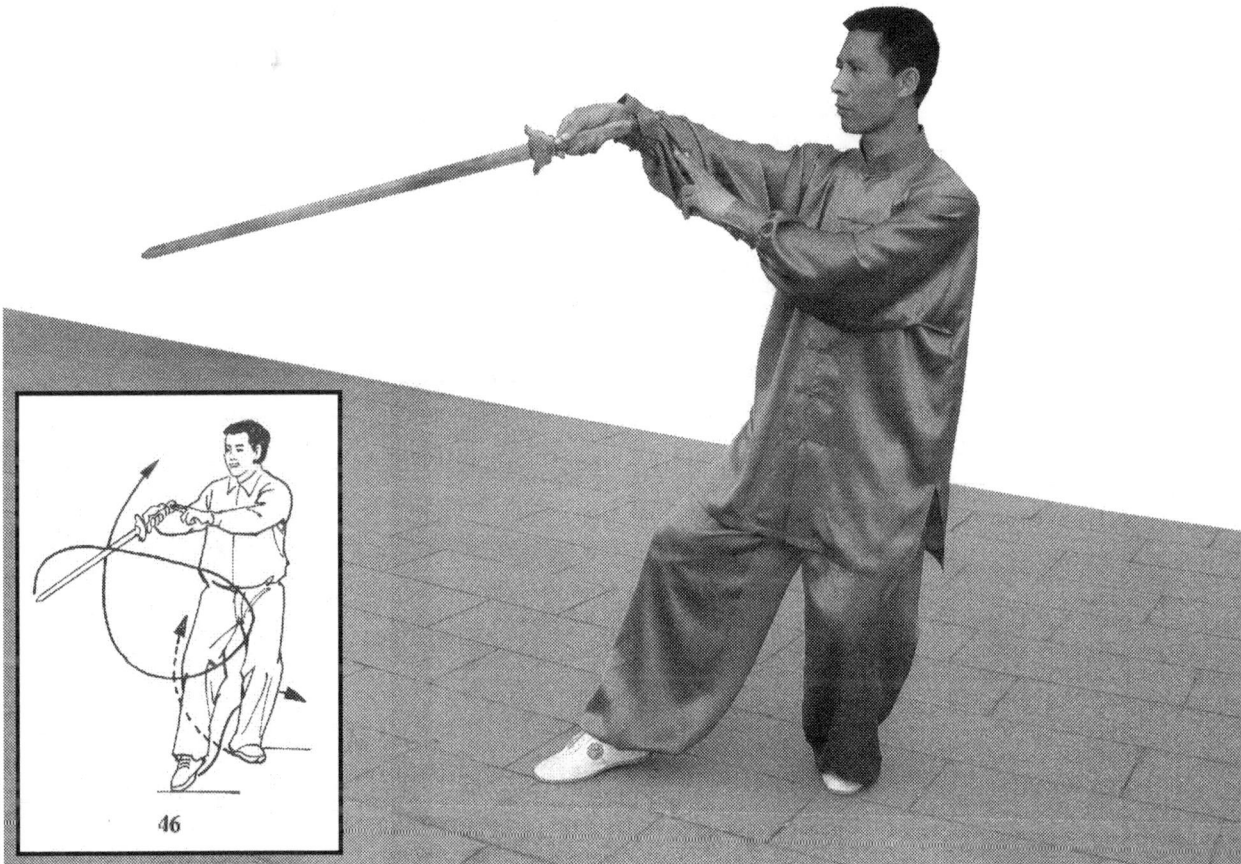

46

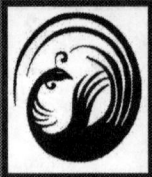

Group Three

The fourth group consists of eight forms shown below.

25. *Hold Sword with One-leg Up*
26. *Hang-up Chop with Right Bow Stance*
27. *Wheel Chop with Empty Stance*
28. *Retreat Step and Attack Backward*
29. *Step Forward and Flat Pierce*
30. *Pull Back Sword with T-Stance*
31. *Rotate and Flat Slice*
32. *Forward Pierce with Left Bow Stance*

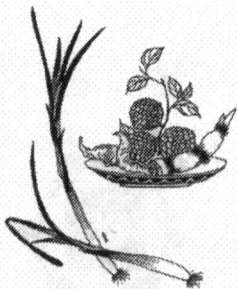

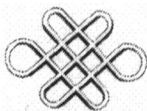

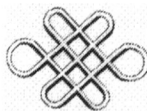

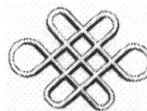

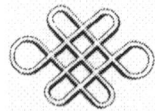

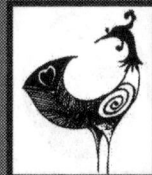

Form 25. Hold Sword with One-leg Up

(47) Lift your right foot backward and shift the center to the right leg. Then stand on the right leg and lift your left knee in an independent stance while circling the sword above your head. Face west (Figure 47).

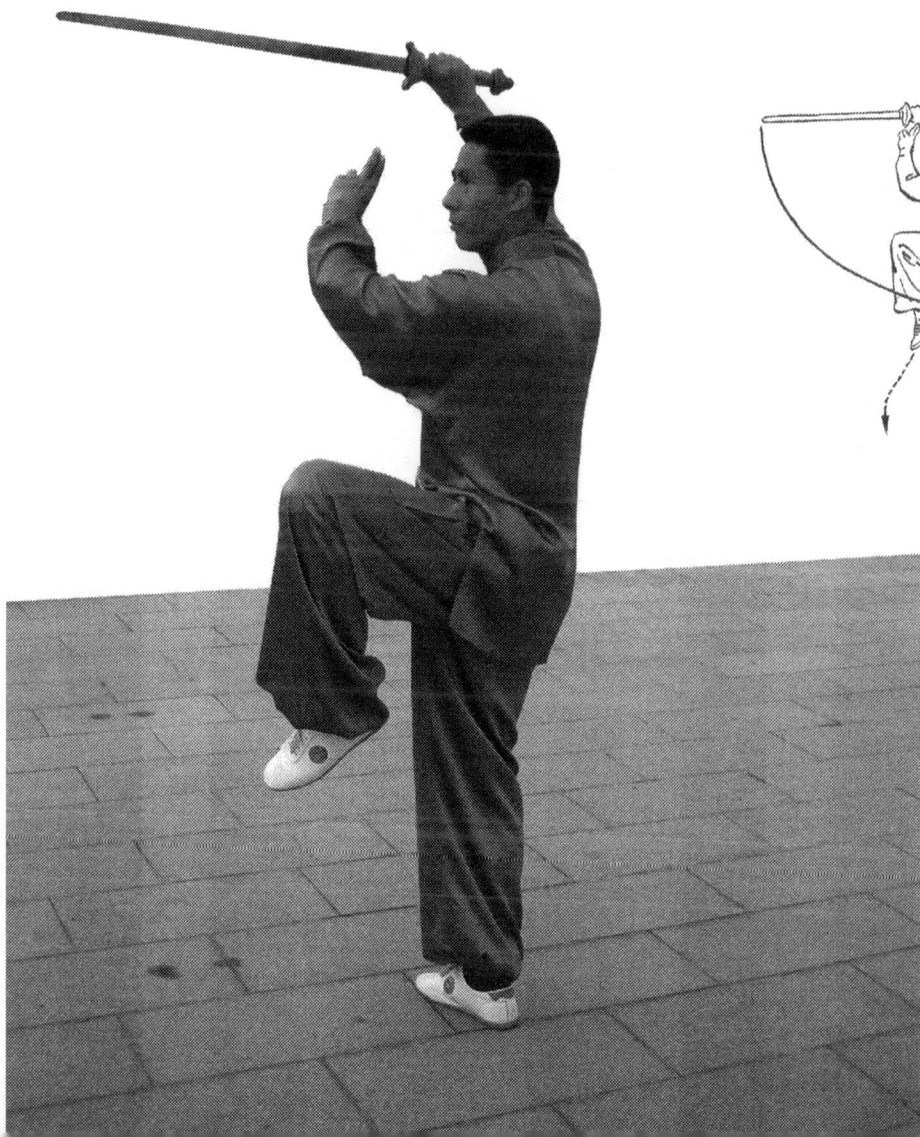

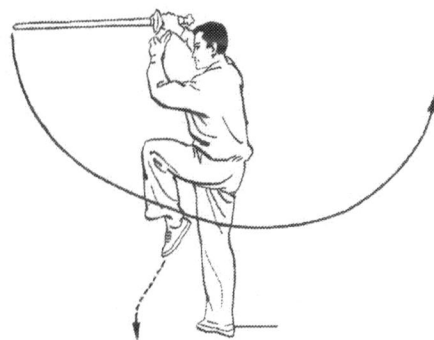

47

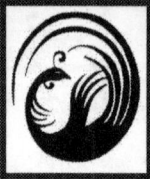
Form 26. Hang-up Chop with Right Bow Stance

(48) Put down your left foot while circling backward the sword to the left side. Face southeast (Figure 48).

(49) Place your right foot forward in a right bow stance while circling the sword forward and chopping. Face west (Figure 49).

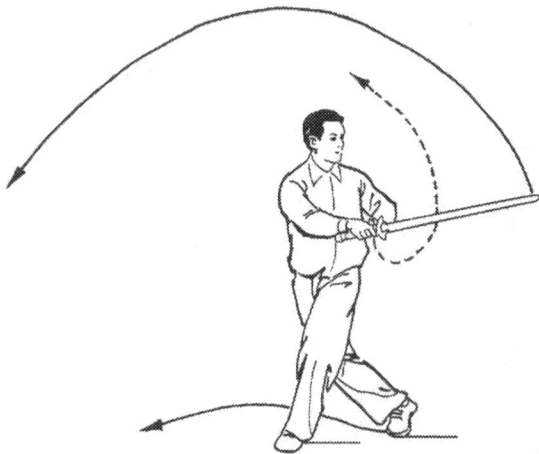

48

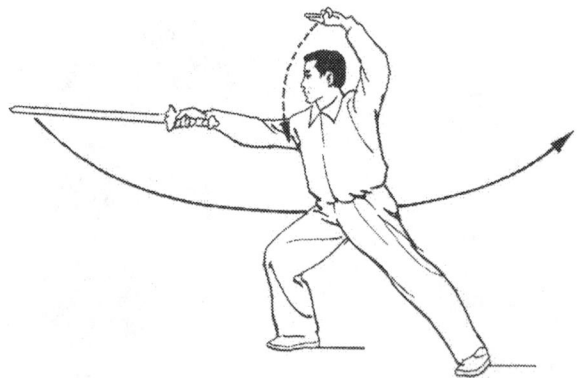

49

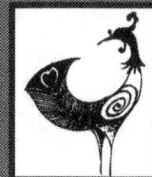

Figure 48. Put down your left foot while circling backward the sword to the left side. Face southeast.

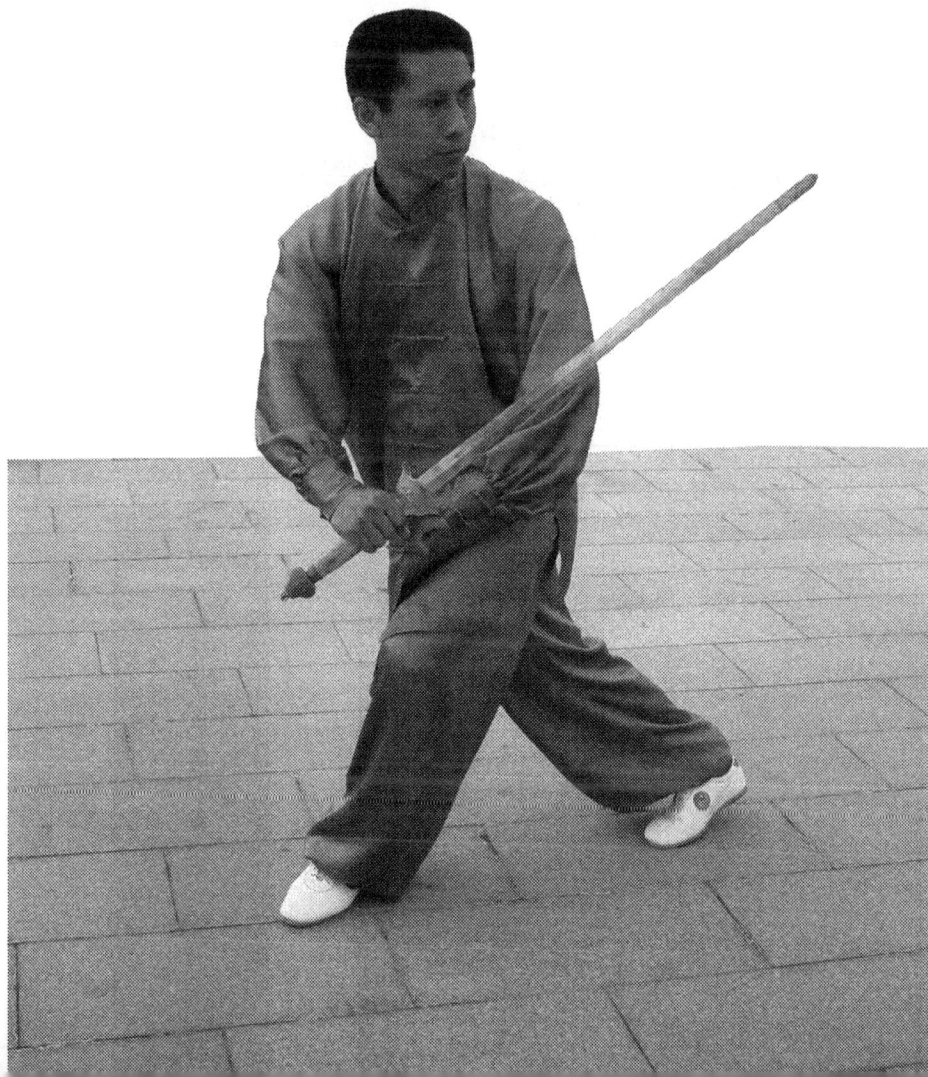

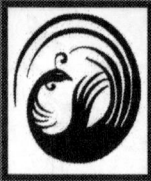

Figure 49. Place your right foot forward in a right bow stance while circling the sword forward and chopping. Face west.

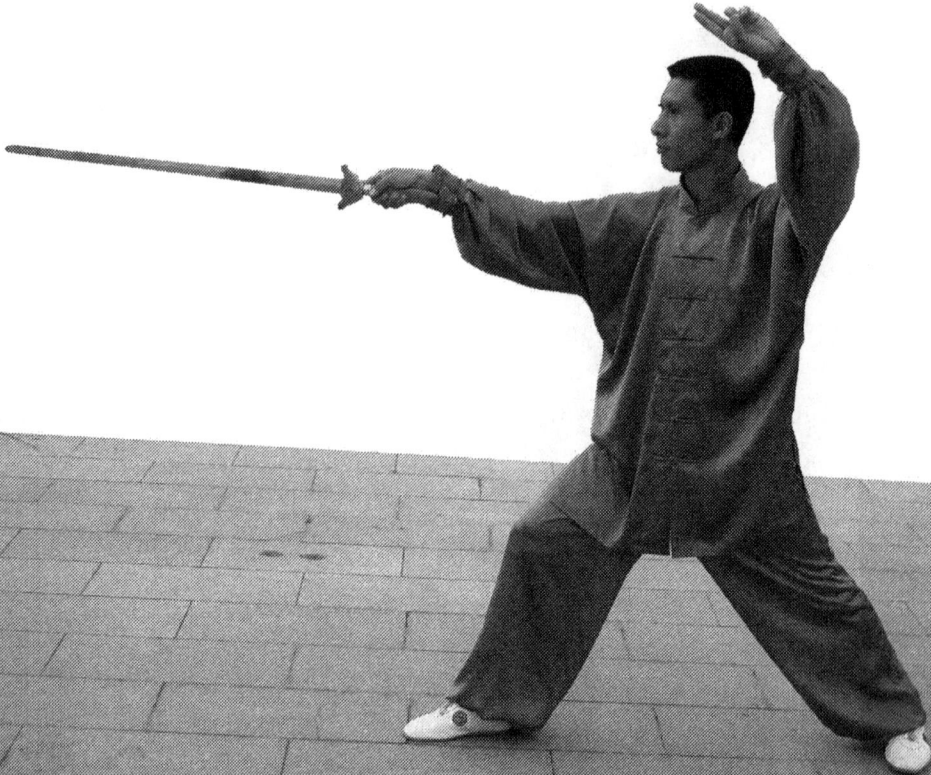

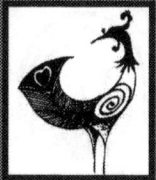

Form 27. Wheel Chop with Empty Stance

(50) Shift your center backward while circling the sword back to the east direction (Figure 50).

(51) Shift your center to the right leg again and place your left foot forward. Then transfer your center to the left leg in a sit-on left empty stance while chopping the sword like a wheel with your right foot in front. Face west (Figure 51).

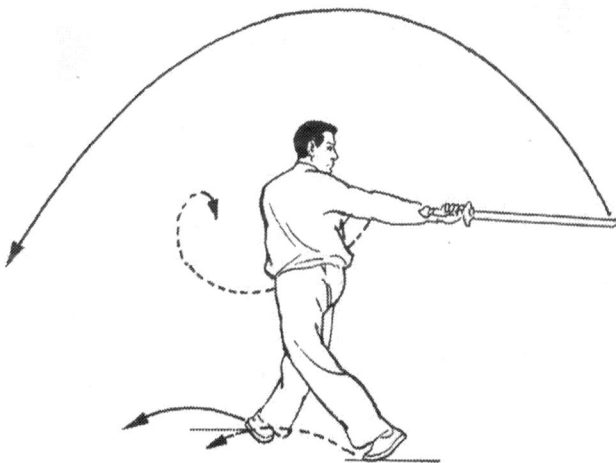

50

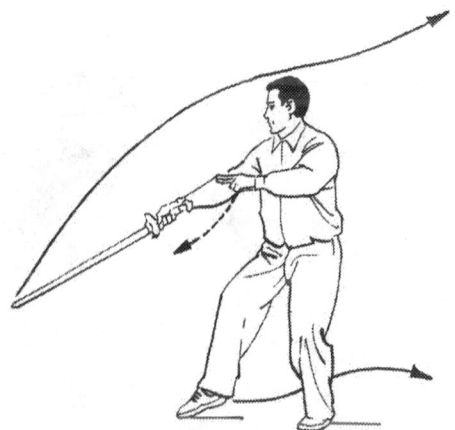

51

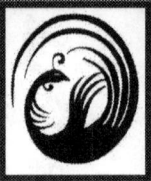

Figure 50. Shift your center backward while circling the sword back to the east direction.

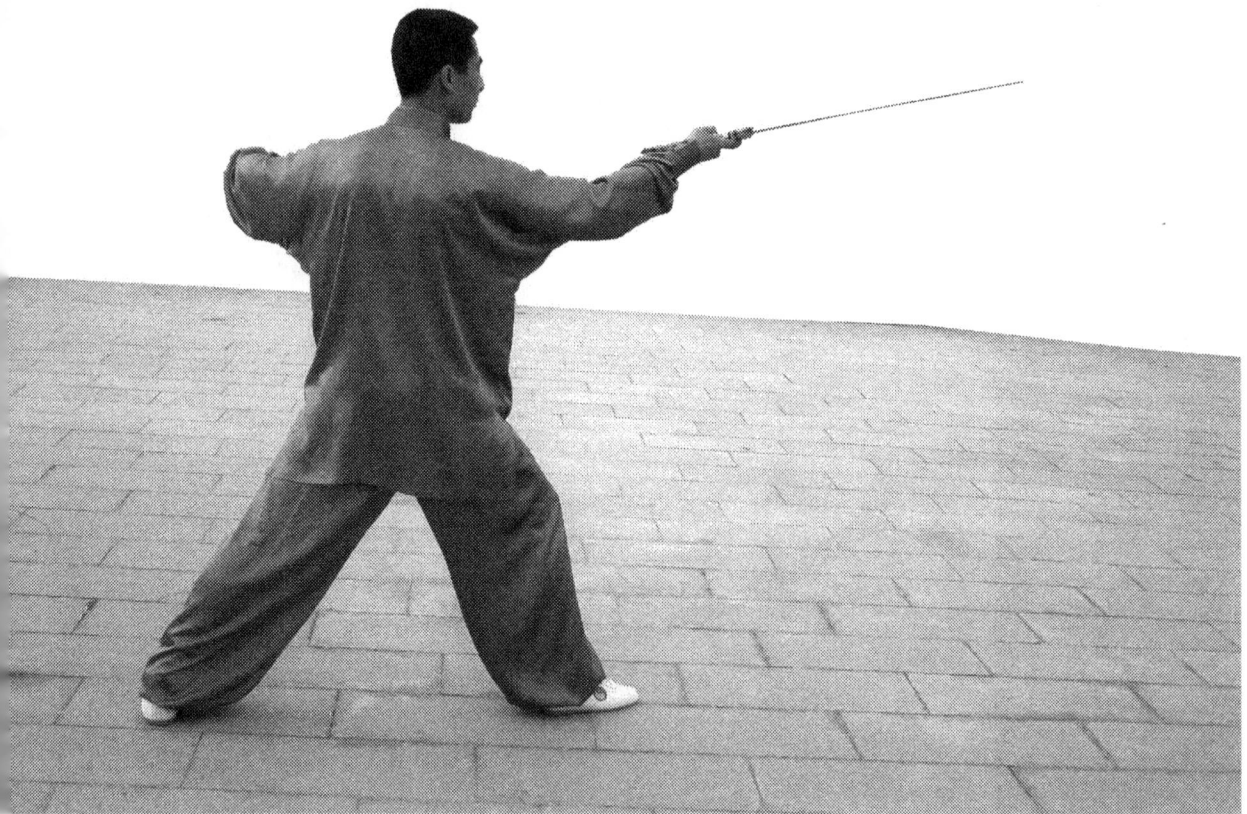

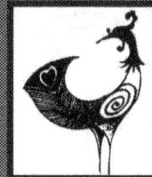

Figure 51. Shift your center to the right leg again and place your left foot forward. Then transfer your center to the left leg in a sit-on left empty stance while chopping the sword like a wheel with your right foot in front. Face west.

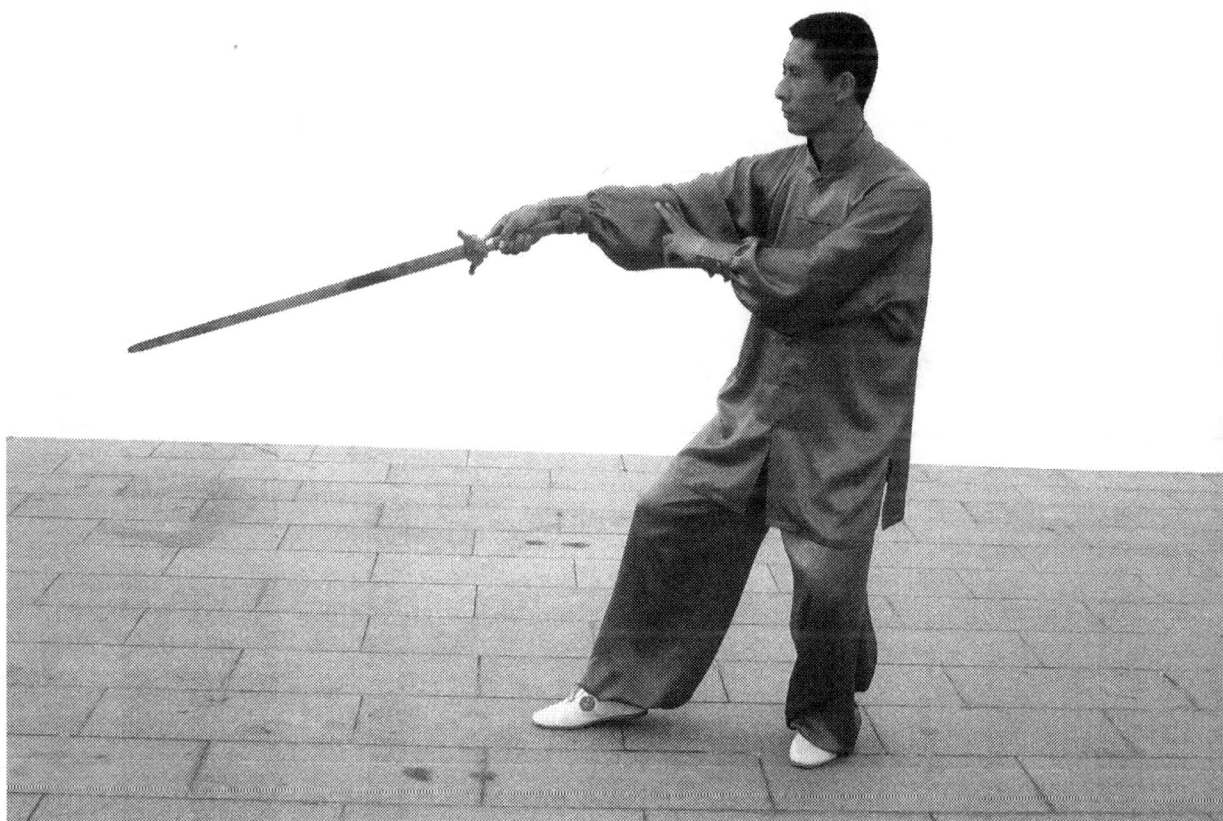

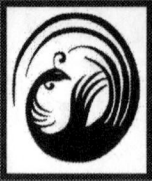

Form 28. Retreat Step and Attack Backward

(52) Step back with the right foot in a right lower bow stance in a diagonal direction, then circle the sword backward and upward, and attack. Face north-east (Figure 52).

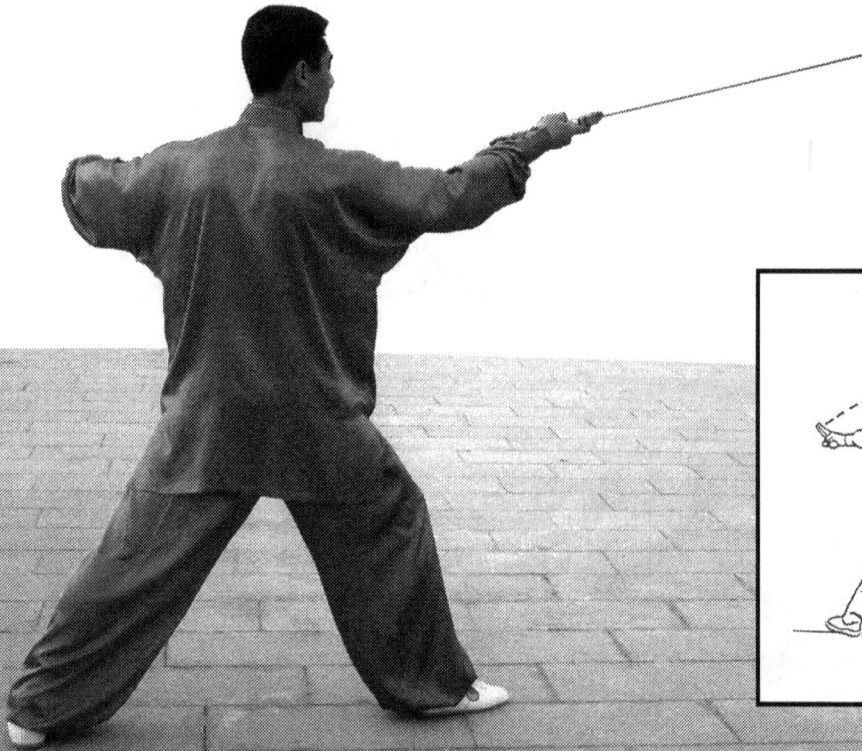

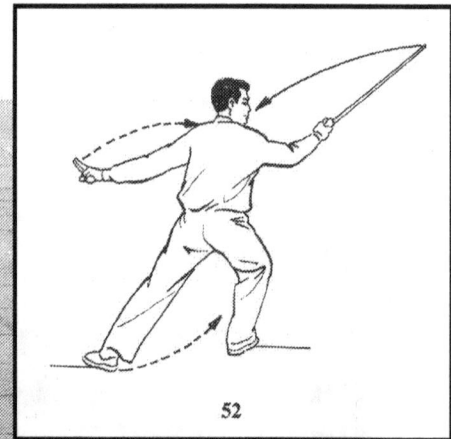

52

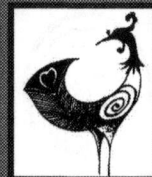

Form 29. Step Forward and Flat Pierce

(53) Stand on your right leg while lifting up your left foot close to the right leg. At the same time, draw the sword and the left hand close to the right side of your body. Face Northeast direction (Figure 53).

(54) Place your left foot forward. Then draw your right foot forward in a right bow stance while piercing the sword forward horizontally. Face west (Figure 54).

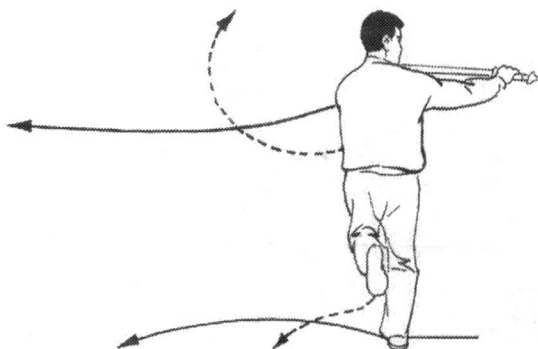

53

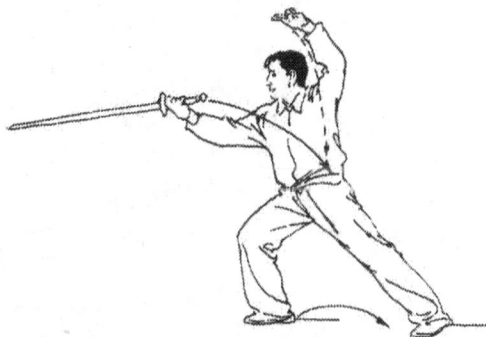

54

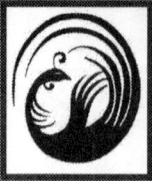

Figure 53. Stand on your right leg while lifting up your left foot close to the right leg. At the same time, draw the sword and the left hand close to the right side of your body. Face Northeast direction.

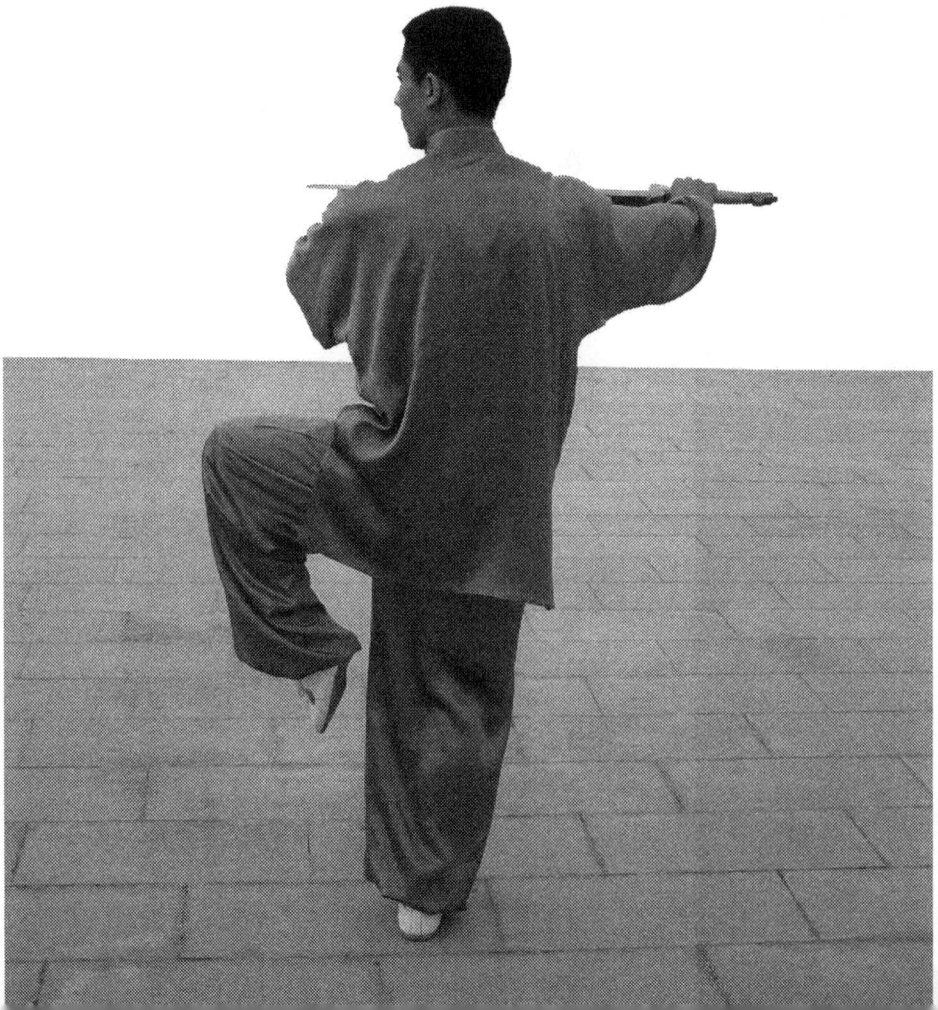

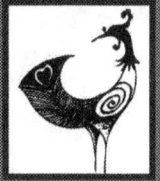

Figure 54. Place your left foot forward. Then draw your right foot forward in a right bow stance while piercing the sword forward horizontally. Face west.

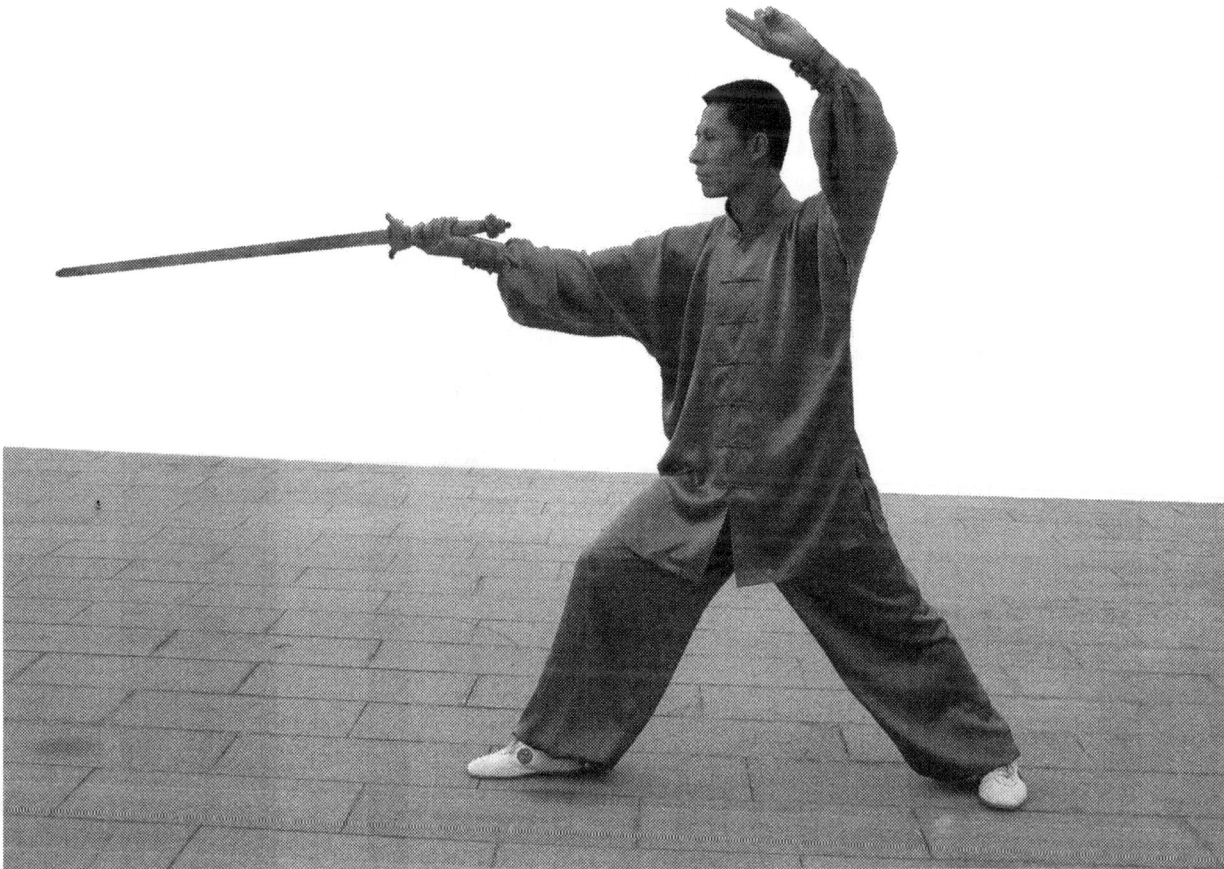

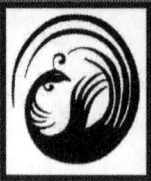

Form 30. Pull Back Sword with T-Stance

(55) Shift your center to the left leg and draw the right foot close to the left foot with the right toe touching the ground while pulling back the sword in front of your chest. Face: southwest (Figure 55).

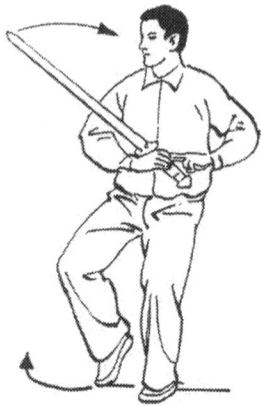

55

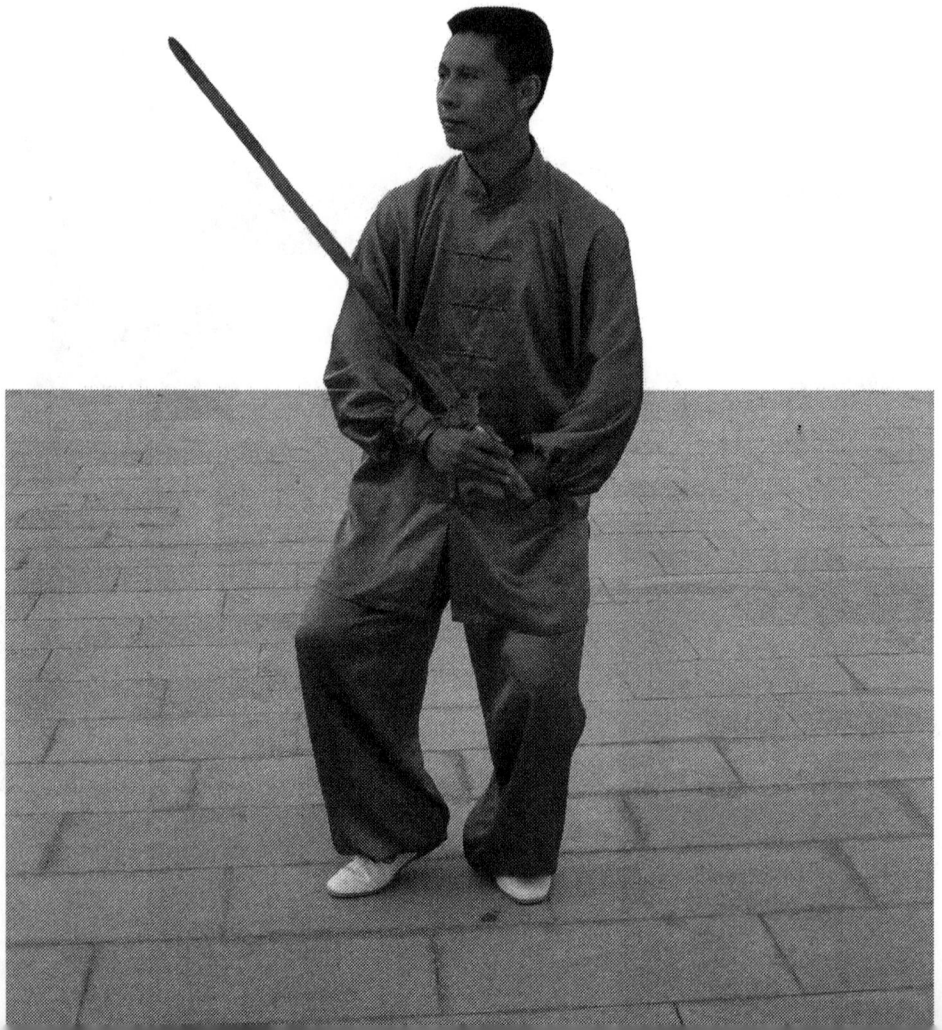

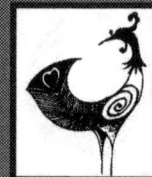

Form 31. Rotate and Flat Slice

(56) Rotate the body and the sword by pivoting on the right heel (Figure 56).

(57) Rotate the body and sword by pivoting on the left heel (Figure 57).

(58) Sit on the right leg in an empty stance with both arms separated. Face south (Figure 58).

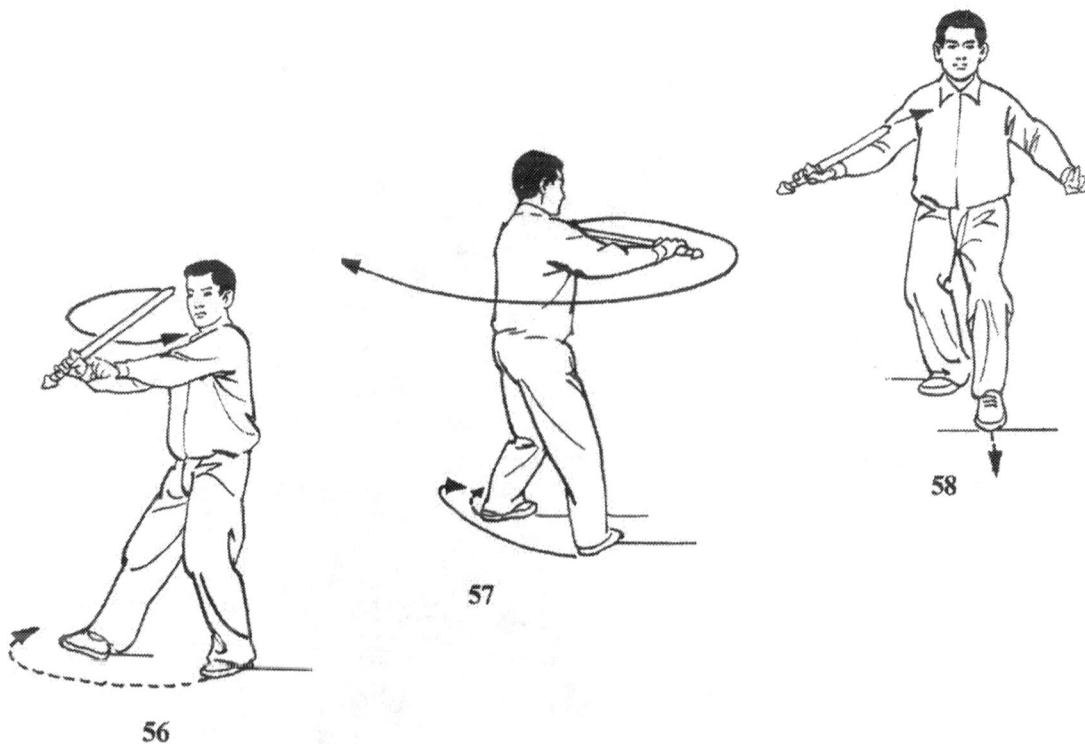

58

57

56

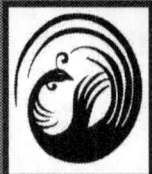

Figure 56. Rotate the body and the sword by pivoting on the right heel.

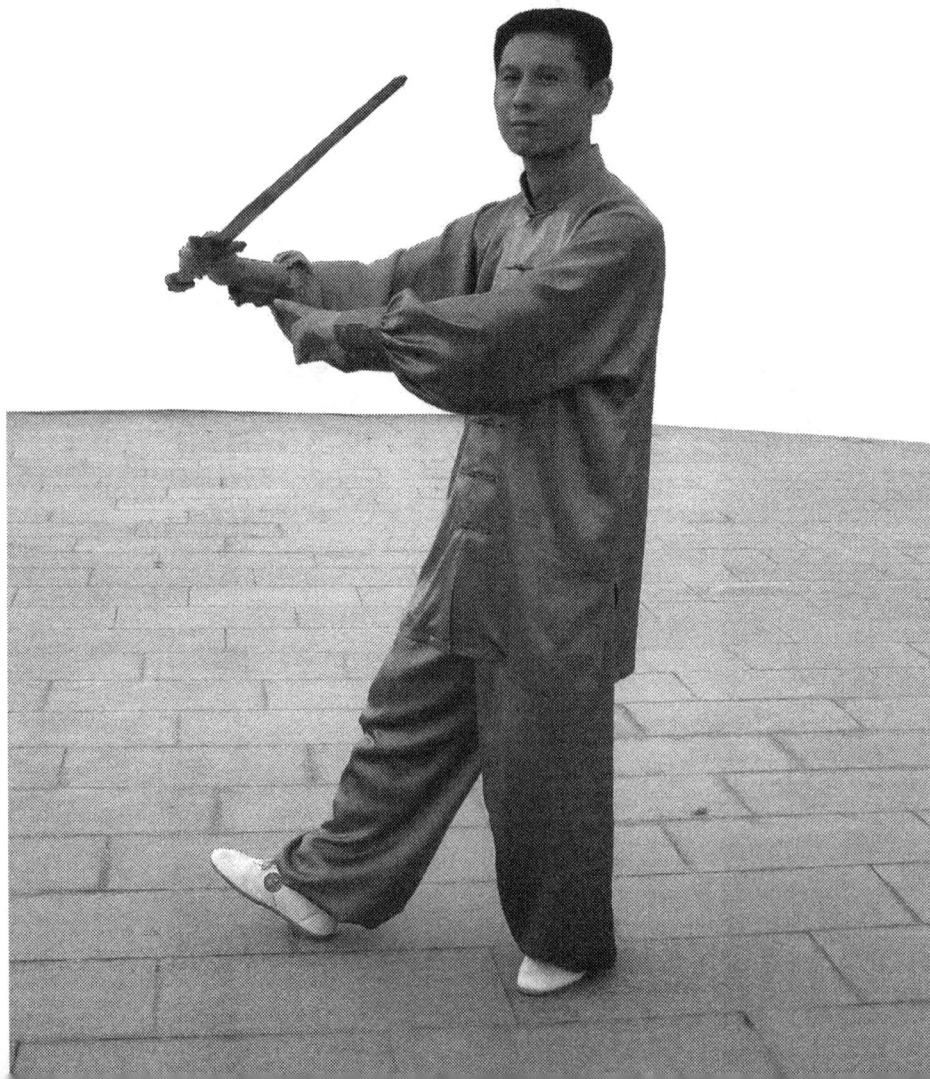

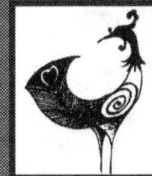

Figure 57. Rotate the body and sword by pivoting on the left heel.

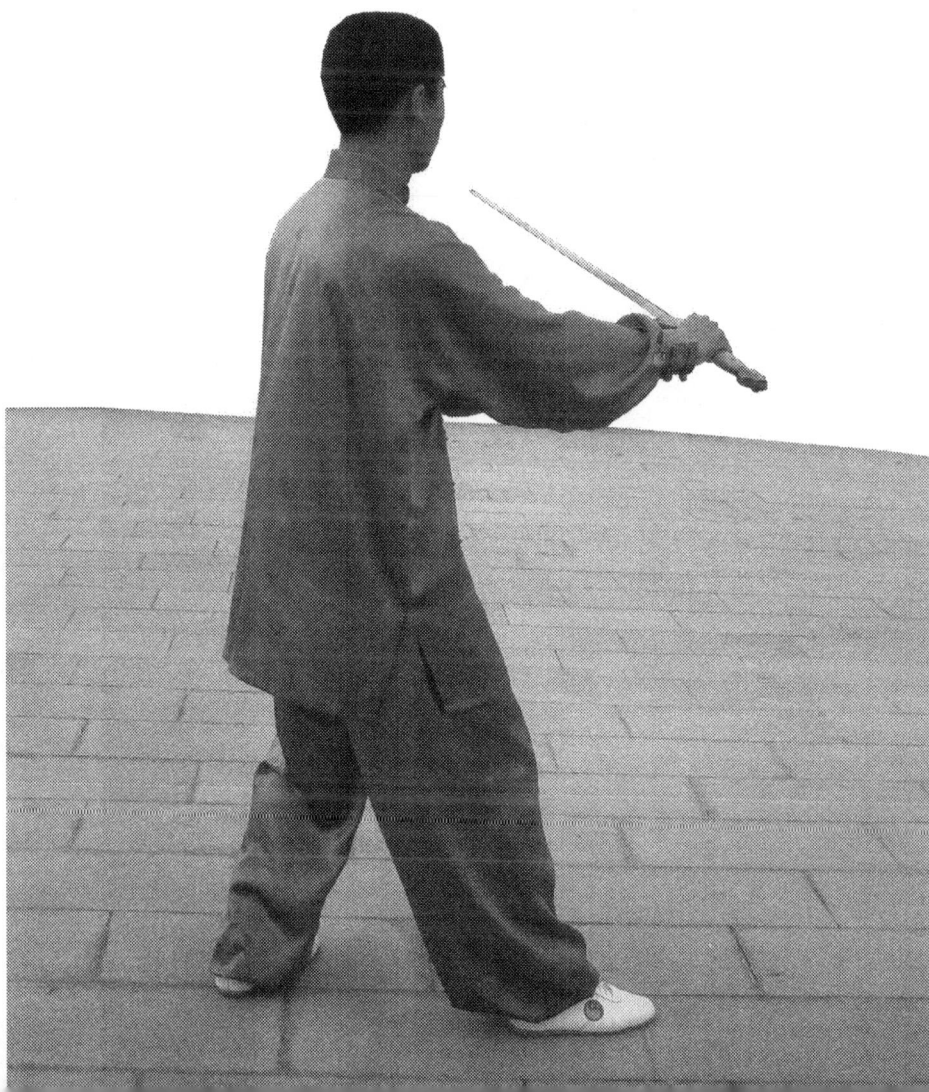

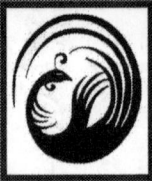

Figure 58. Sit on the right leg in an empty stance with both arms separated. Face south.

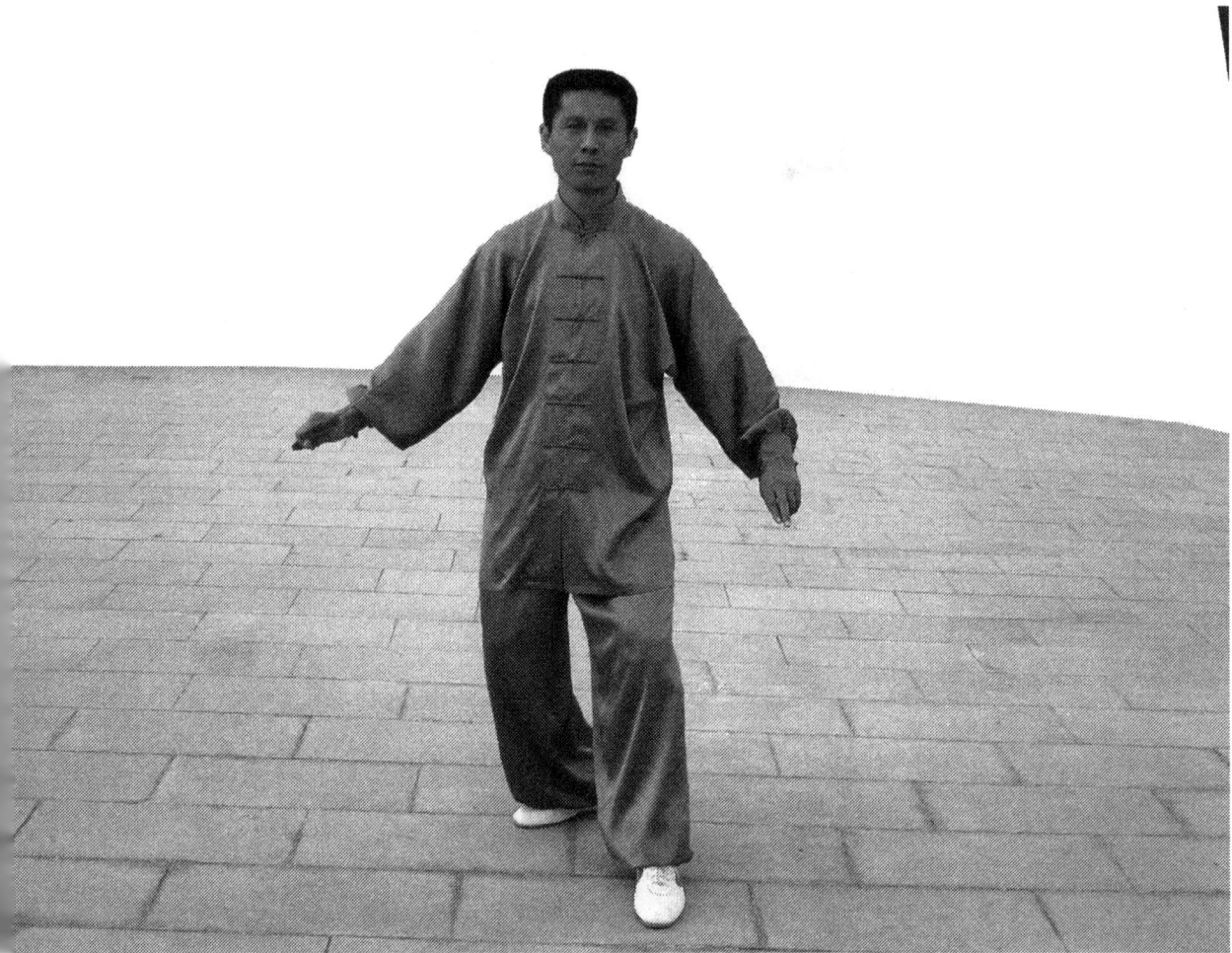

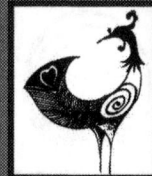

Form 32. Forward Pierce with Left Bow Stance

(59) Change to left bow stance with the left foot forward and pierce the sword forward. Face south (Figure 59).

(60) Shift the center back to your right leg while pulling the sword beside the chest. Face west (Figure 60).

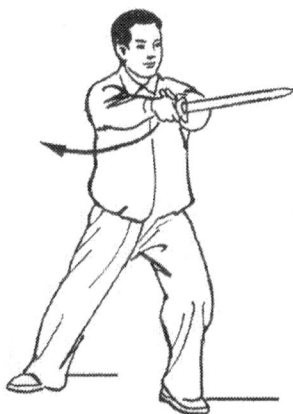

59

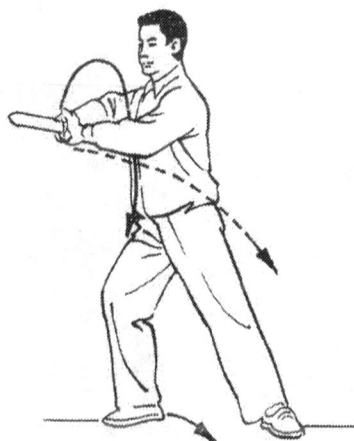

60

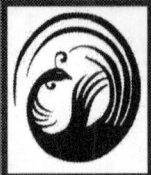

Figure 59. Change to left bow stance with the left foot forward and pierce the sword forward. Face south.

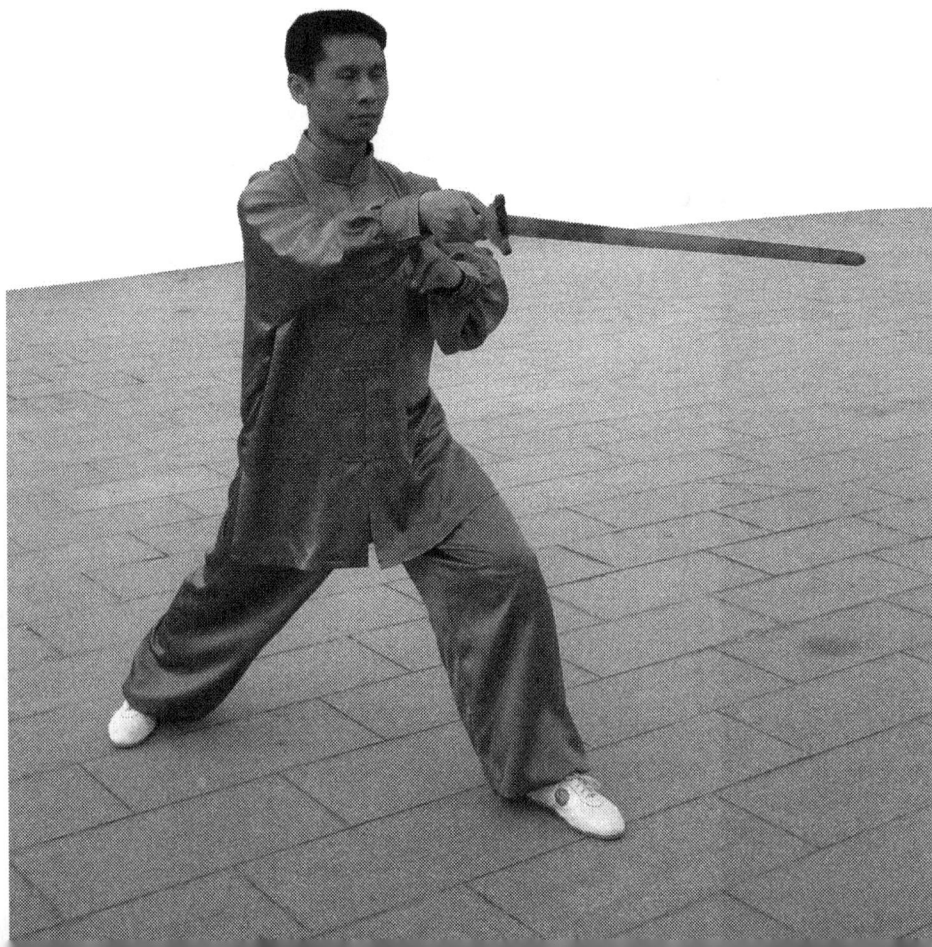

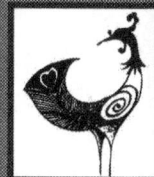

Figure 60. Shift the center back to your right leg while pulling the sword beside the chest. Face west.

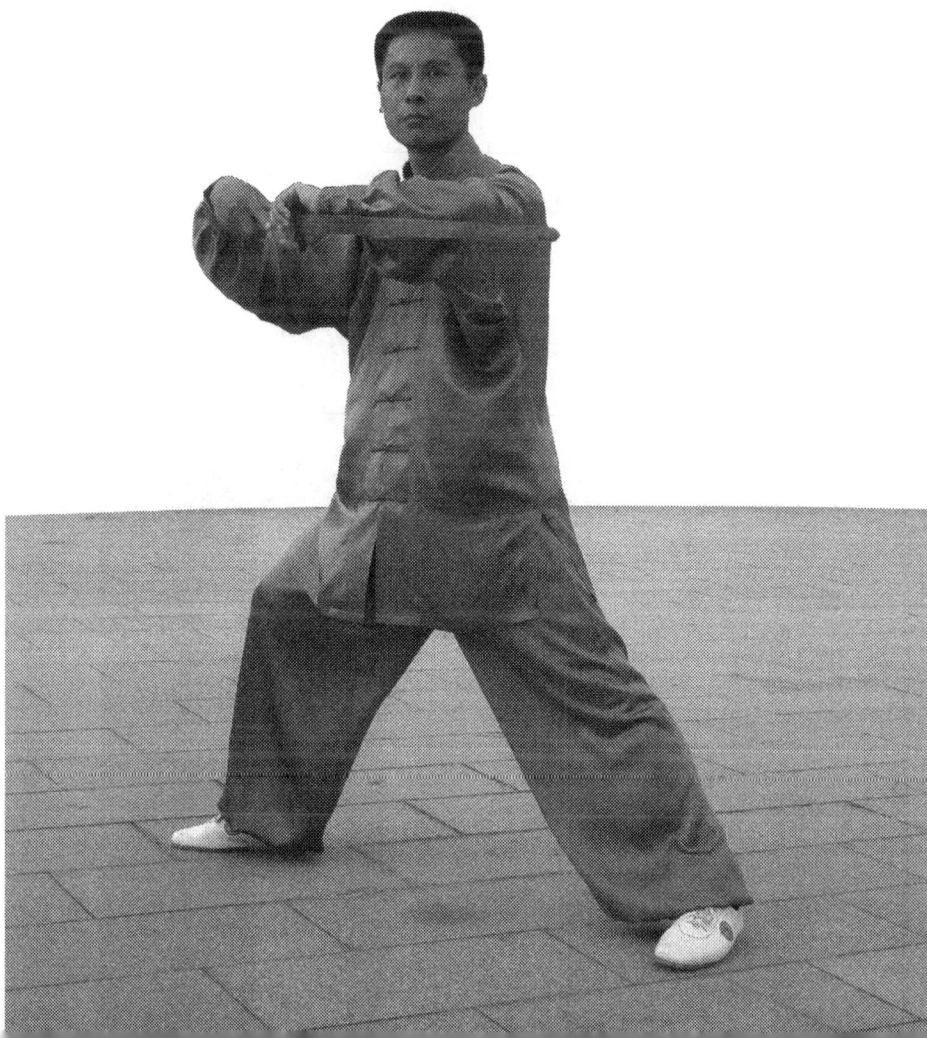

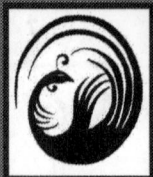

Closing Form

(61) Shift the center forward to your left leg and draw your right foot close to your left foot about shoulder width apart while changing the sword from the right hand to the left hand. Both arms are naturally sinking back with the sword up.

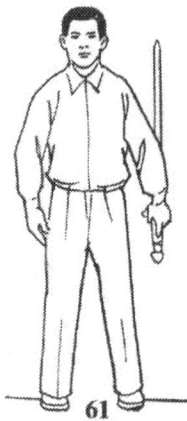

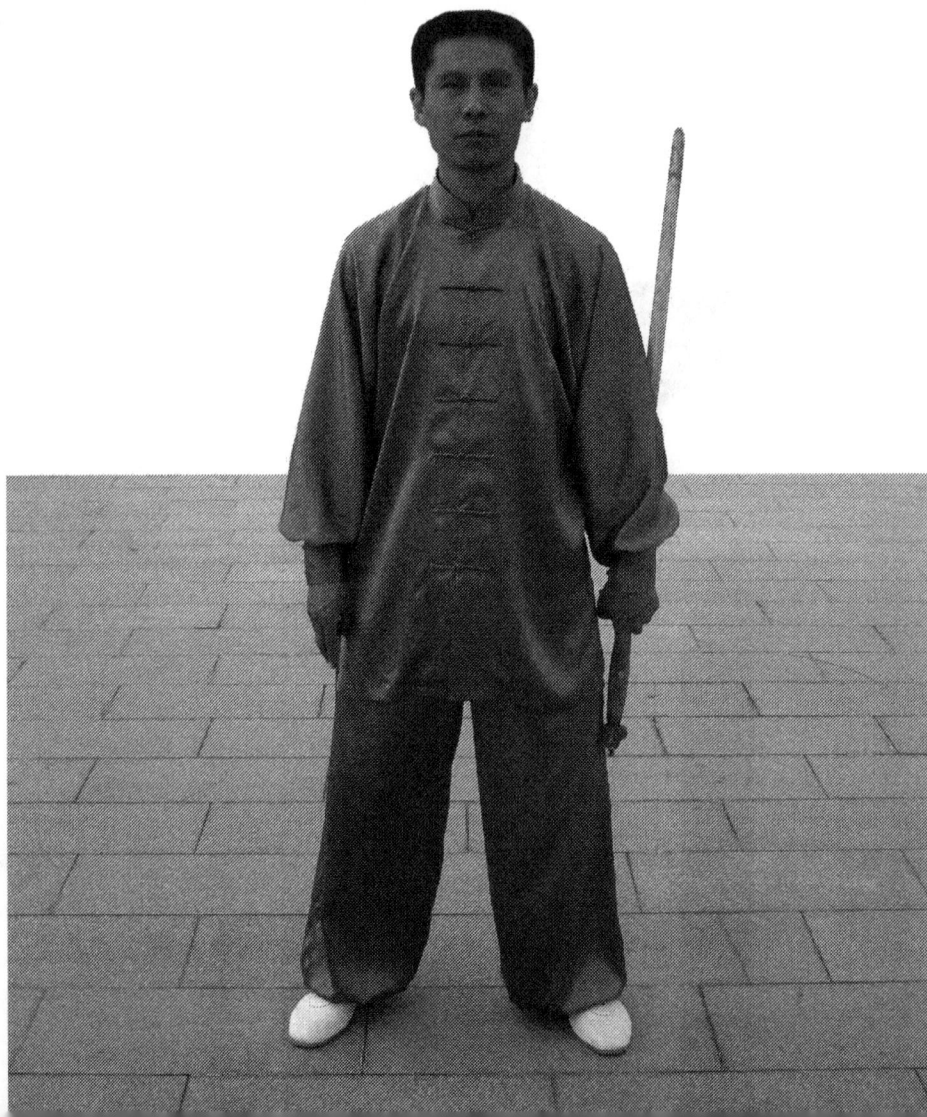

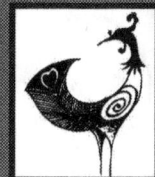

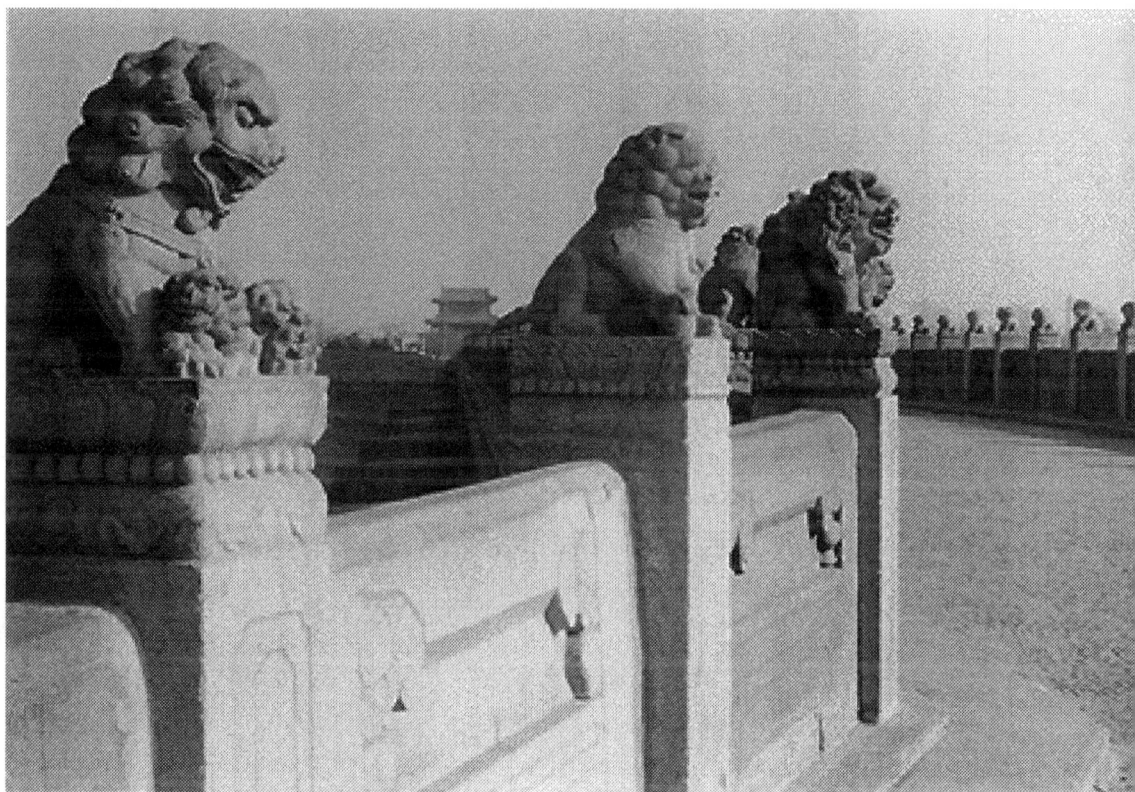

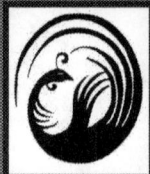

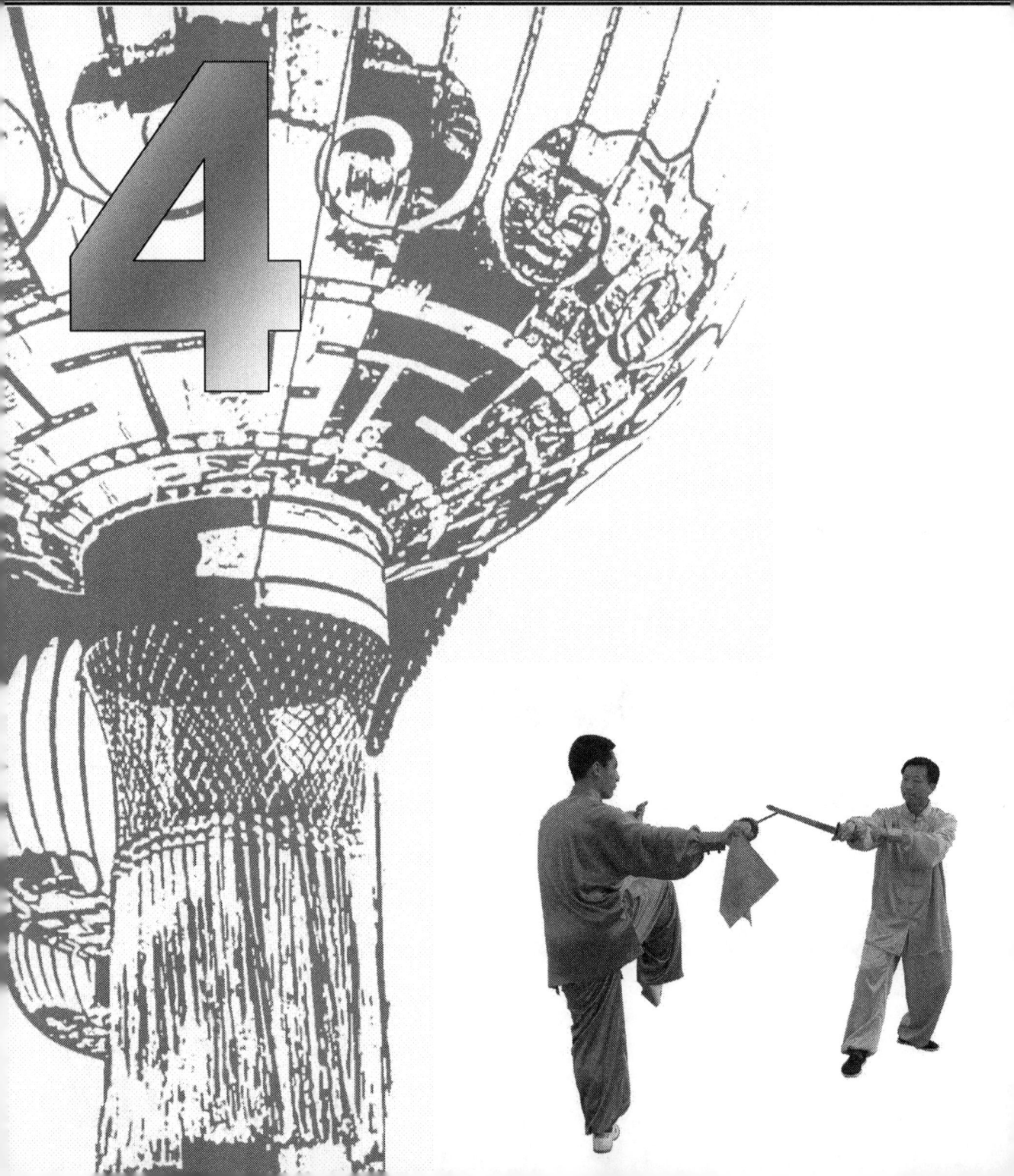

4

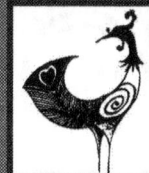

Chapter 4: Principles of Tai Chi

If we compare Tai Chi to other forms of martial arts or physical exercises, it does not emphasize on building power and muscular force. Rather, Tai Chi teaches a person how to use soft movements and smooth blending of energy to achieve a goal, whether the goal is to dissolve an attacking force or simply to improve health and fitness. Tai Chi first became noted as a combat art when it was brought to Beijing, the capital of China, by Yang Lu Chan in 1820. The martial art of Tai Chi is based on the concepts of the Yin and Yang, as is true for the fitness programs of Tai Chi. In ancient Chinese philosophy, Yin and Yang exist in both spiritual and material states. Tai Chi uses Yin and Yang Theory to guide its practice. For example, "Part when moving; Merge when in stillness." Tai Chi is soft and sticky. Martial artists of Tai Chi stick to attackers to gain the same speed as the attacking force rather than block or directly resist the coming force. According to the classical Tai Chi works, "Respond rapid

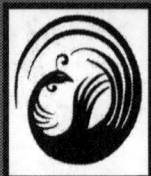

moves with speed; Follow the slow moves with slow moves."
These core concepts are used to guide and form the physical
moves of Tai Chi.

The basic principles of Yang style are:

- Relaxation
- Separation of Yin and Yang (substantial and insubstantial)
- All moments are directed and commanded by the waist
- The spine is kept straight and upright
- A focused awareness of slowness, gracefulness, softness, relaxation, and keeping a flowing continuity when executing the forms.

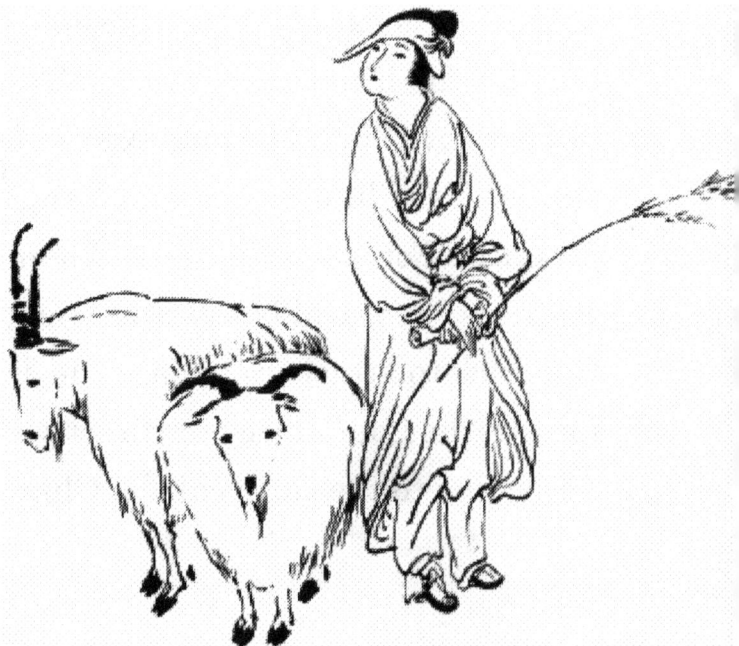

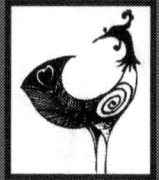

The Theoretical Foundations of Tai Chi

1.   Foundation in Martial Art

Tai Chi originally is a pure form of martial art. It has its own unique fighting principles and attacking power. Here the fighting principle means that every move of Tai Chi has an intent of offense and defense and is coherent with the its fighting philosophy. Tai Chi on the battlefield has real effects in overcoming the enemy and is essentially different from gymnastics and dancing. For sure, Tai Chi is not dancing.

From its origination to the later development, Tai Chi borrowed techniques from many other martial arts and absorbed the best of them. According to Chinese history record, in the Ming dynasty, the famous warrior Qi Ji Guang developed a powerful form of boxing and wrote a book called "The bible of 32 forms of Chuan". A later study shows that there were many similarities between Tai Chi Chuan and Qi's Chuan in terms of the forms, postures and the sequence of moves. Some scholars even claimed that Tai Chi was originated from Hong Dong Flash Arm Chuan. Despite the validity of such a claim, Tai Chi has evidently borrowed

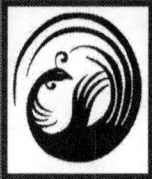

techniques from other martial art forms.

Tai Chi's theoretical foundation is solid. There exist more than 140 articles about the principles and applications of Tai Chi over the last 800 years. From these books and articles, we can easily see the thoughts, techniques, methods and applications of Tai Chi Chuan in combat. For example, in "The Theory of Tai Chi" the author states "Let go when the opponent is hard; Stick to it when following a retreating opponent," which is evidently the Tai Chi's strategy of fighting an enemy. Other examples are "Beat Hand Tips", "Tips of Thirteen Forms" and "Four Word Secrets", which all talked about martial art strategies and techniques.

The modern development of Tai Chi is mainly headed toward the arena of health and fitness. From the viewpoint of sport, it is an excellent exercise used for health benefits, but in forms of martial art. Through its martial art form, it will help people to improve health and fitness; without it, it would not be Tai Chi anymore.

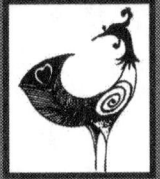

2.   Philosophical Foundation

Tai Chi is steeped in ancient Chinese philosophies, specifically those from Taoism, which is profound and thought-provoking. From the perspective of philosophical background, Tai Chi qualifies to be called "Philosophical Chuan" or Philosophical Fist. Indeed, the philosophies of Taoism are deeply rooted in Tai Chi, guiding every move of it and affecting the strategies in both battlefield and exercise room. The ancient philosophy and Tai Chi movement have combined into a unity, formed a unique form of sport, and created health benefits that are otherwise impossible.

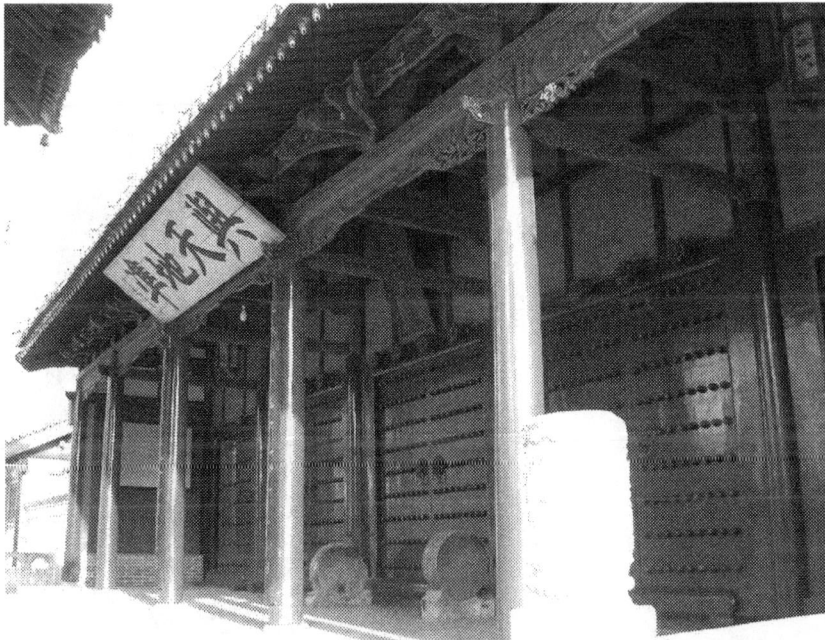

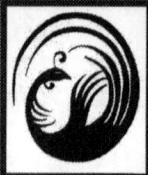

3.   The Foundation from Chinese Medicine

Tai Chi belongs to the inner style of Gongfu. It absorbed the Qi and the theory of acupuncture point network from Chinese traditional medical practice. Its mechanism for health improvement is also based on the Chinese medical theory. By moving all the body parts, Tai Chi practice helps open up all channels inside the body and breaks down the blockage of the Qi. Stretching your body, moving the Qi, and massaging joints are important parts of improving health and increasing strength in Tai Chi practice. The rhythm of breathing in Tai Chi shall be coordinated with the body movements. This is called moving with Qi. Tai Chi also emphasizes the impact of mind on the Tai Chi movements. It says that mind shall follow the forms and the forms shall not separate from the mind. It is believed in Tai Chi that the lack of intent inside will result in insufficient release of energy outside.

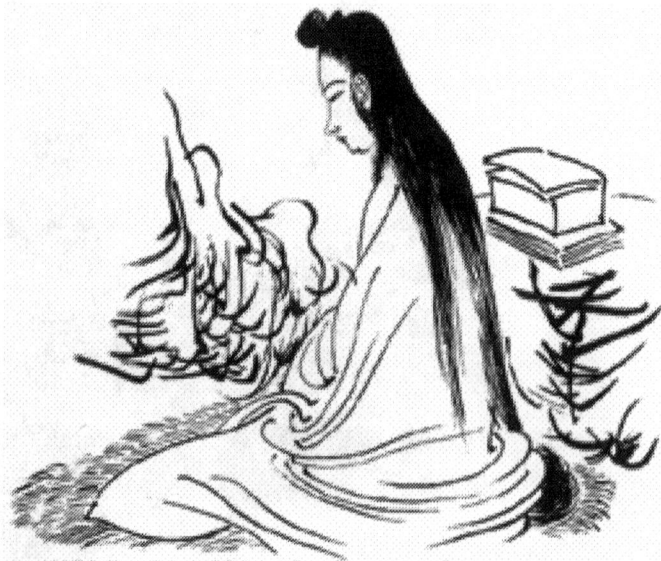

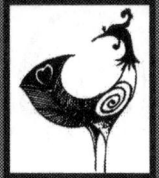

The Sword and Its Characteristics

The sword has been used as one of the primary weapons in China for thousands of years and is called the king of weapons by those who love the grace of the swordsmanship. In ancient China, the sword is used as a combat weapon for officers and legendary warriors. The sword has double edges for cutting and a sharp tip for piercing. It is lethal and agile in practice and permits graceful movements than heavy weight weapons. In China, the sword is played like the swimming dragon, which is thought to be scholarly and graceful. For many, the sword is used for defense rather than attack. Some times, sword is used for warrior dance, in which the sword is not just a weapon for the performing warrior but also a decorative tool to display his dancing skills. As time goes by, sword now plays little combat roles and has no military value. Rather, it becomes a toll for fitness exercises originated from martial arts. In the same time, the size and weight of the sword have been modified to suit this purpose.

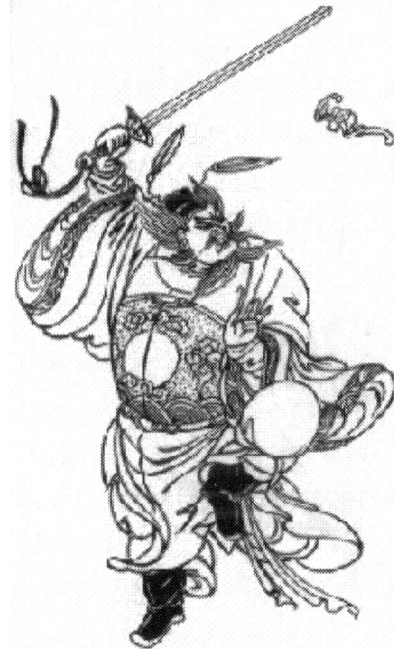

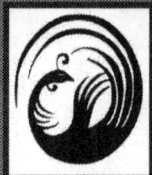

Orientations:

In performing these 32 sword forms, you should imagine you are standing in the middle of a compass. You are facing south. North side is directly behind you. To your right is west and to your left is east. Southwest is halfway between south and west. Southeast is halfway between south and east. Northwest is halfway between north and west. And northeast is halfway between north and east. Although your position will change as you move through the Forms, these directions will remain fixed. Keep these directions in your mind. It will help to align your movements and master Tai Chi Sword effectively.

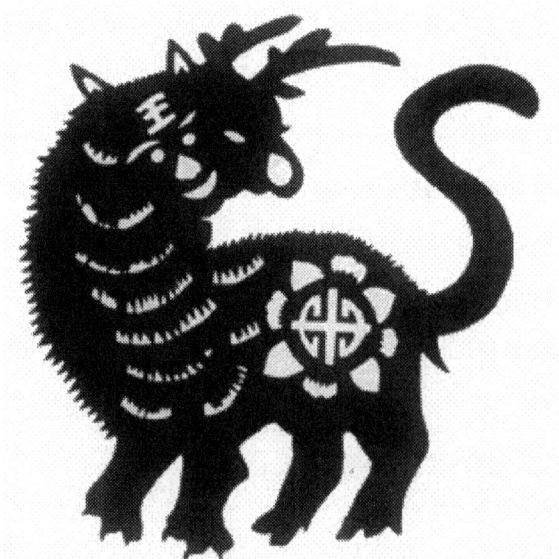

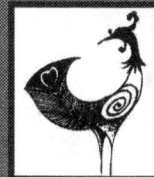
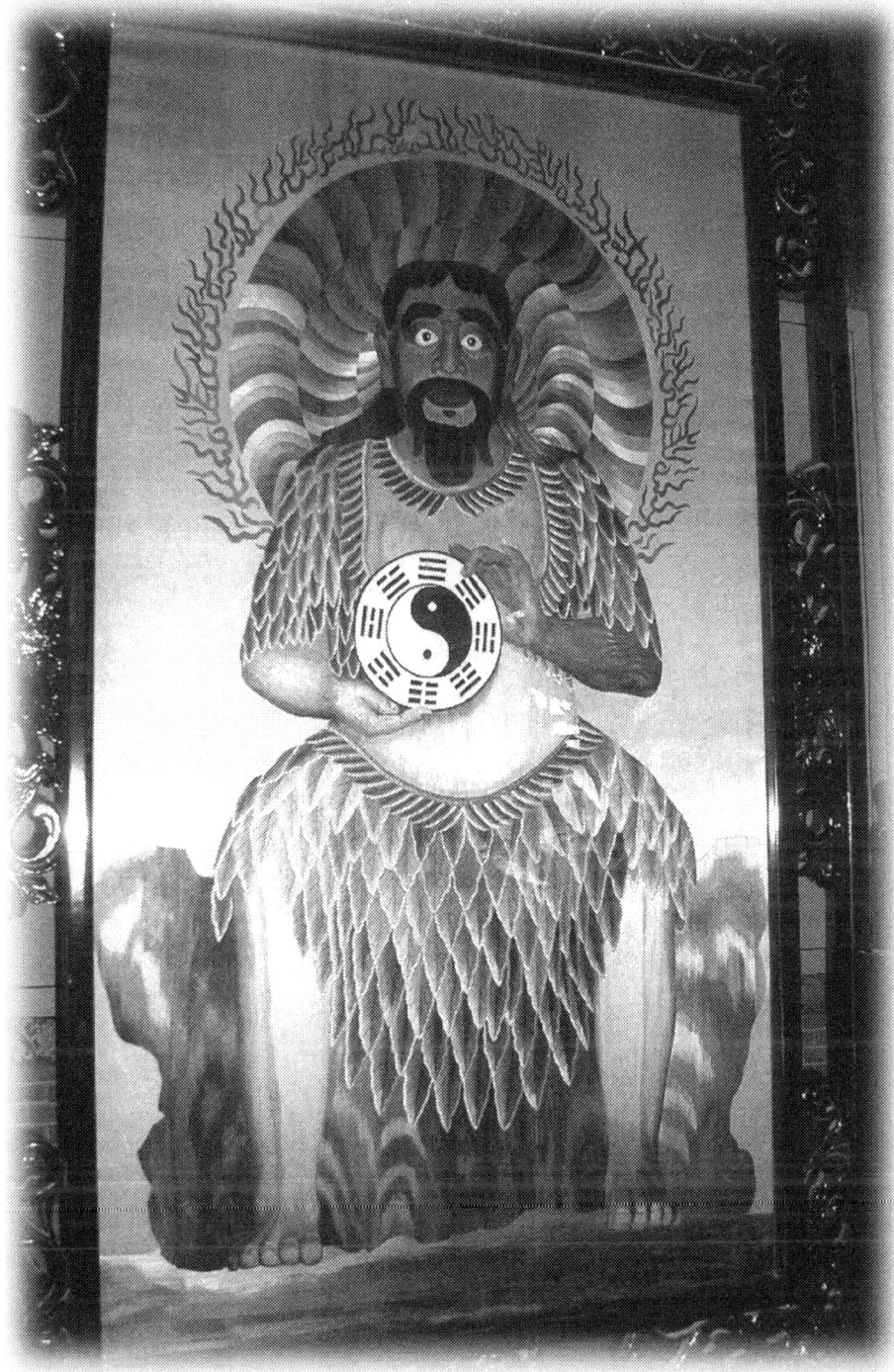

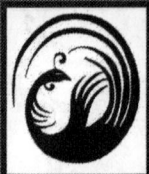

The Transitions between Sword Forms

Beginning Form

In the beginning of this form, you face south. After rotations, your body faces east at the end of this form.

1. Form 1:

In this form, you face east.

2. Form 2

In this form, you step back with rotation to the right side and then turn and face east side with an independent stance on the right leg.

3. Form 3

After rotation, you face east side with the left bow stance.

4. Form 4

After rotation, you face east side with the right bow stance.

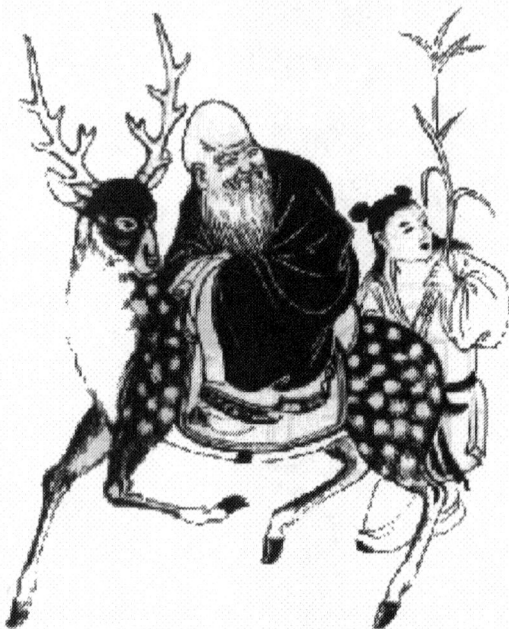

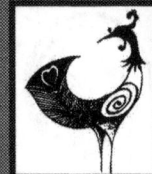

5. Form 5

After rotation, you face east side with the left bow stance.

6. Form 6

After rotation, you face east side and look downward with an independent stance on the right leg.

7. Form 7

In this form you sit back on the left leg and face northeast.

8. Form 8

With an forward step and an independent stance on the right leg, you face east and upward.

9. Form 9

In this form you slice the sword downward and look east side and downward.

10. Form 10

You pierce the sword in the northeast direction and face northeast.

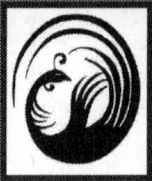

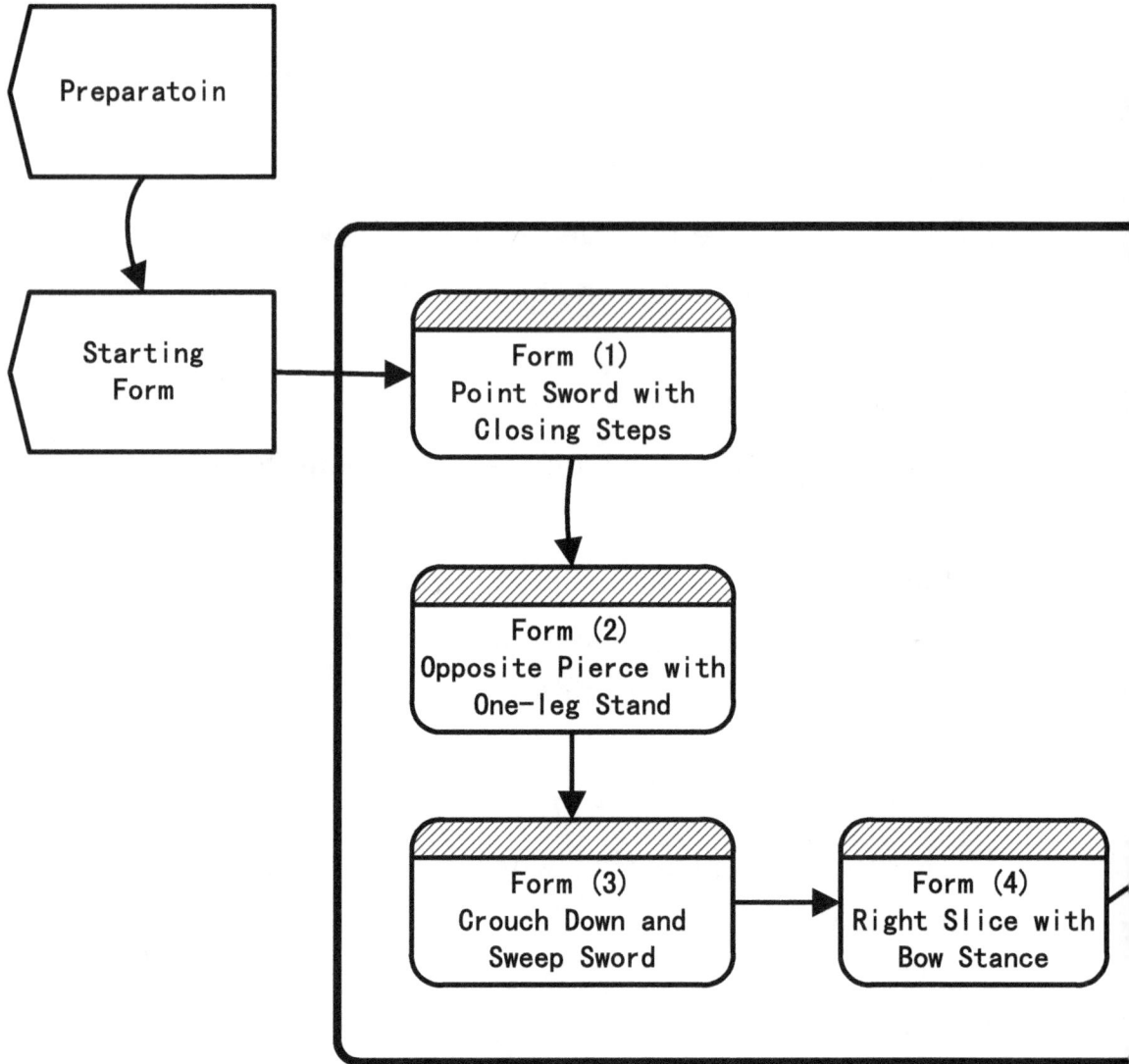

Preparatoin

Starting
Form

Form (1)
Point Sword with
Closing Steps

Form (2)
Opposite Pierce with
One-leg Stand

Form (3)
Crouch Down and
Sweep Sword

Form (4)
Right Slice with
Bow Stance

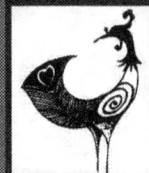

Group One
Transitions

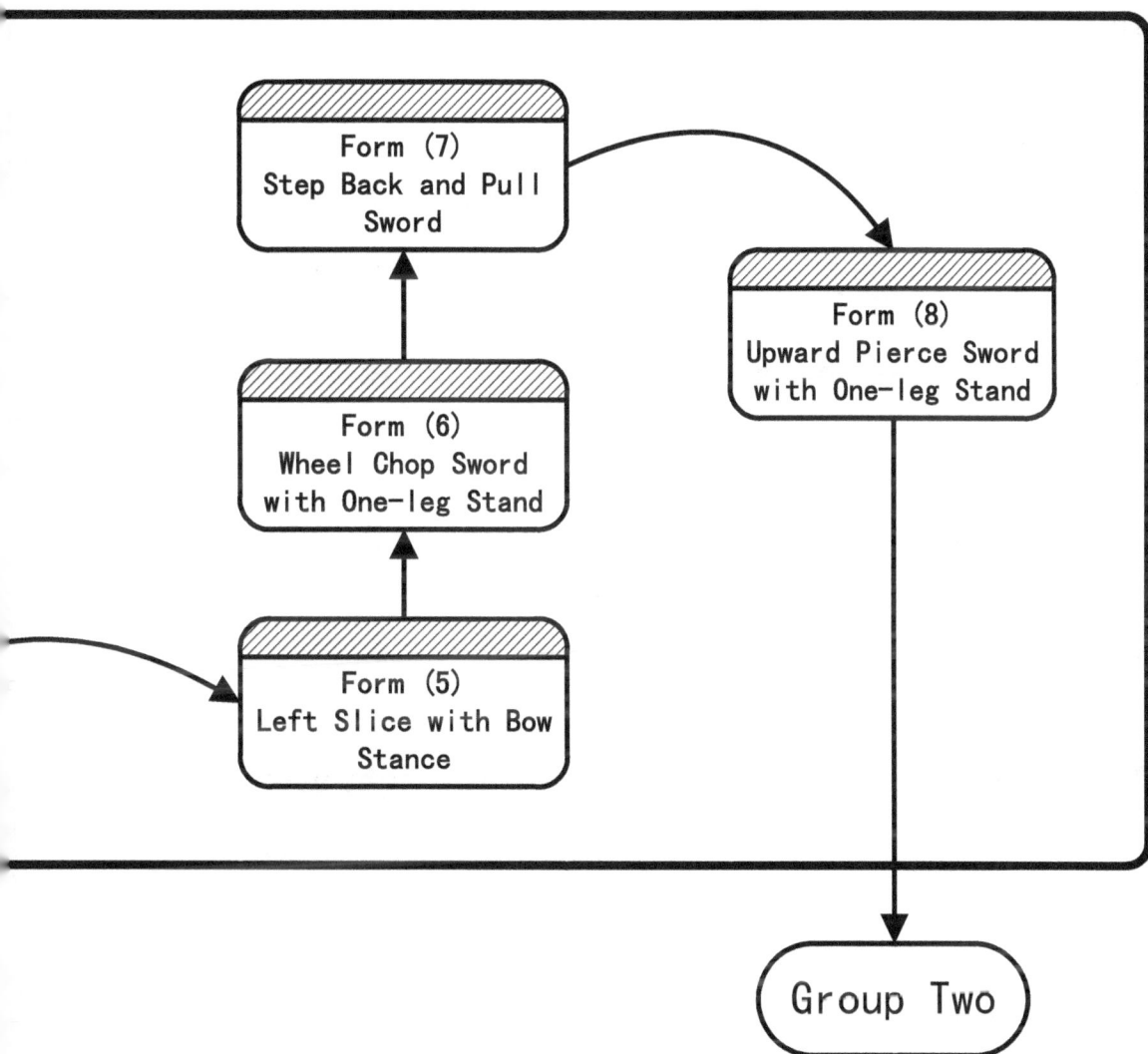

Form (7)
Step Back and Pull
Sword

Form (8)
Upward Pierce Sword
with One-leg Stand

Form (6)
Wheel Chop Sword
with One-leg Stand

Form (5)
Left Slice with Bow
Stance

Group Two

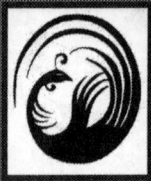

11. Form 11

With a 270 degree rotation, you face northwest.

12. Form 12

In this form you sit on the right leg and face to west.

13. Form 13

You hold up your sword to the west.

14. Form 14

In this form you jump and pierce the sword to the west.

15. Form 15

In this form you turn your body and sit on an empty stance to the west.

16. Form 16

You swing your sword to the west with the right bow stance.

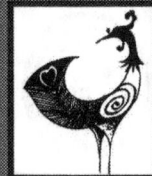

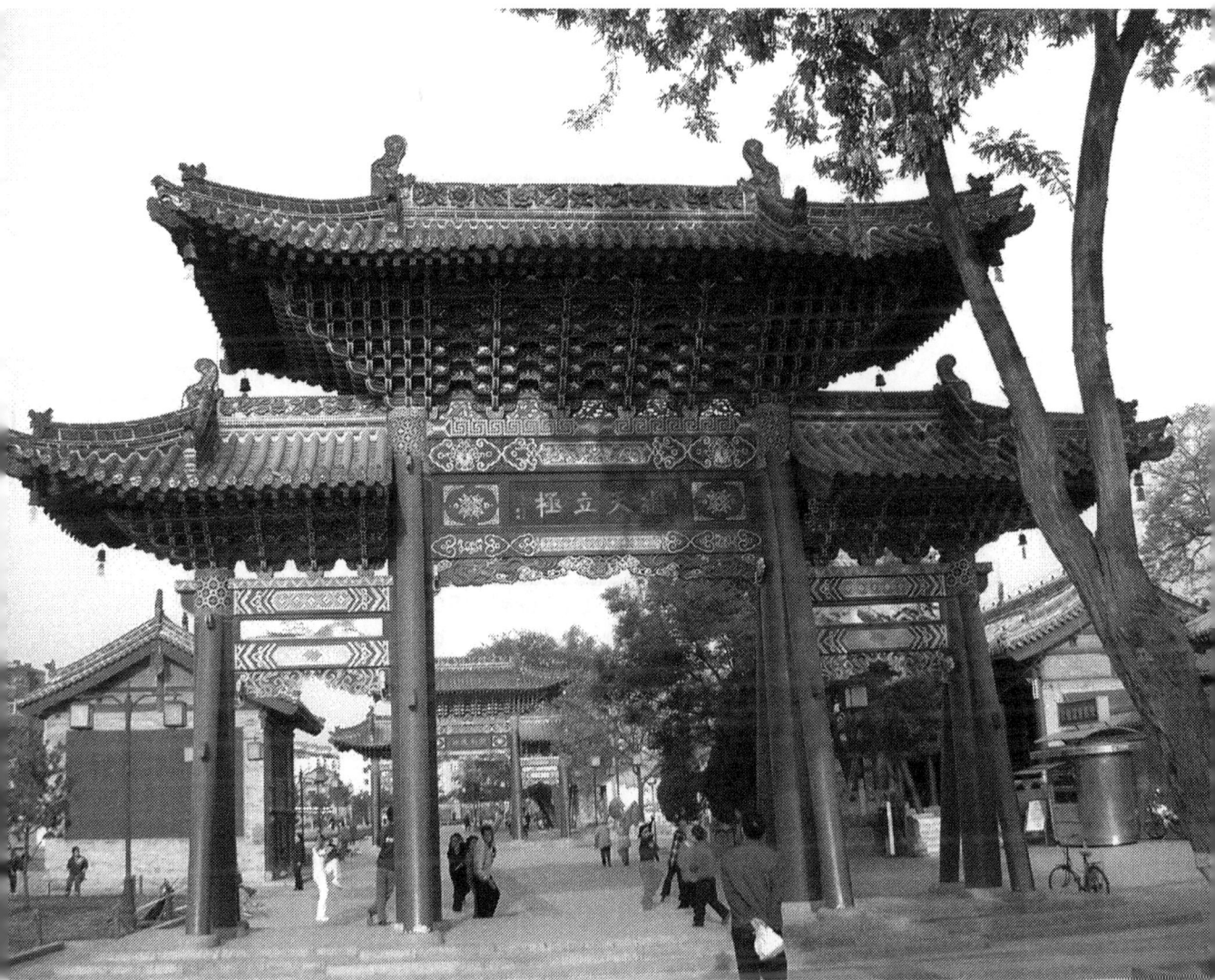

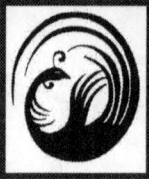

Group Two

Transitions

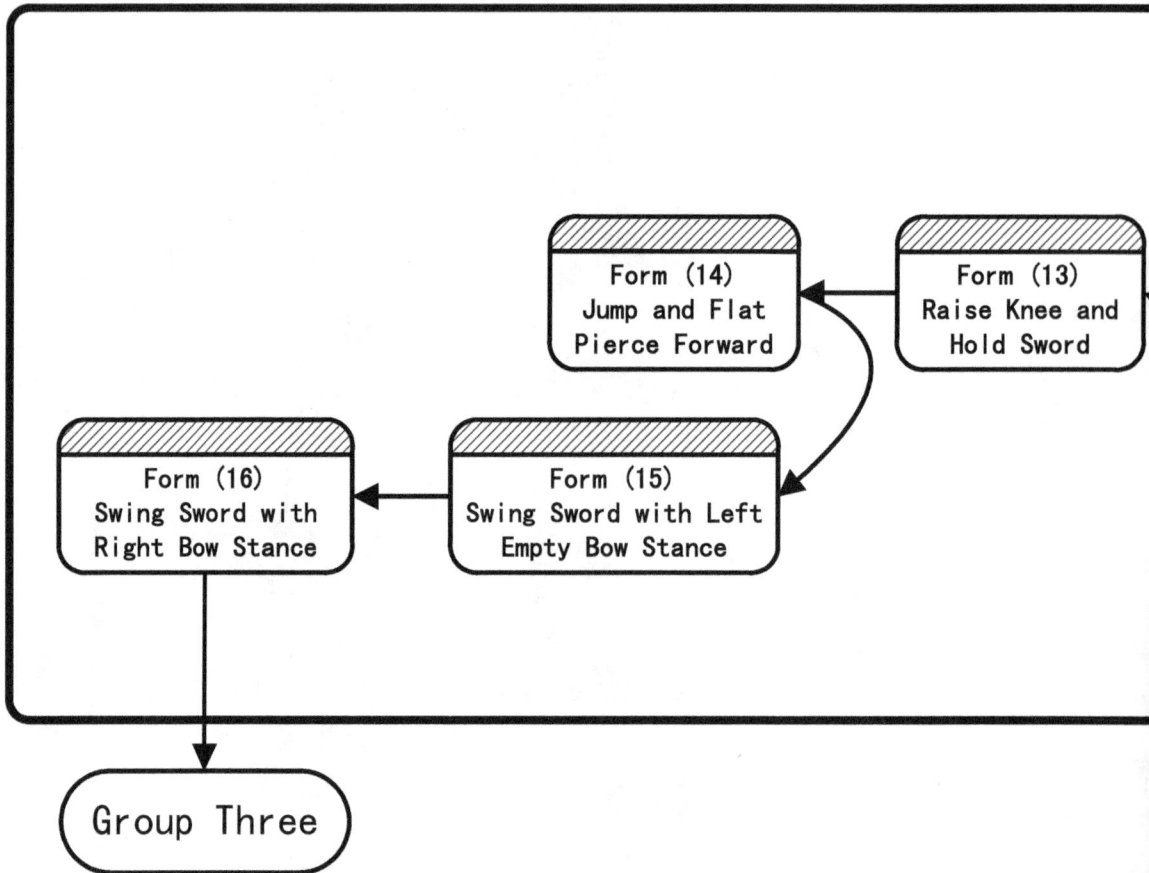

Form (14) Jump and Flat Pierce Forward	Form (13) Raise Knee and Hold Sword
Form (16) Swing Sword with Right Bow Stance	Form (15) Swing Sword with Left Empty Bow Stance

Group Three

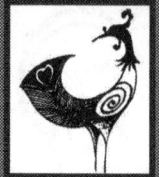

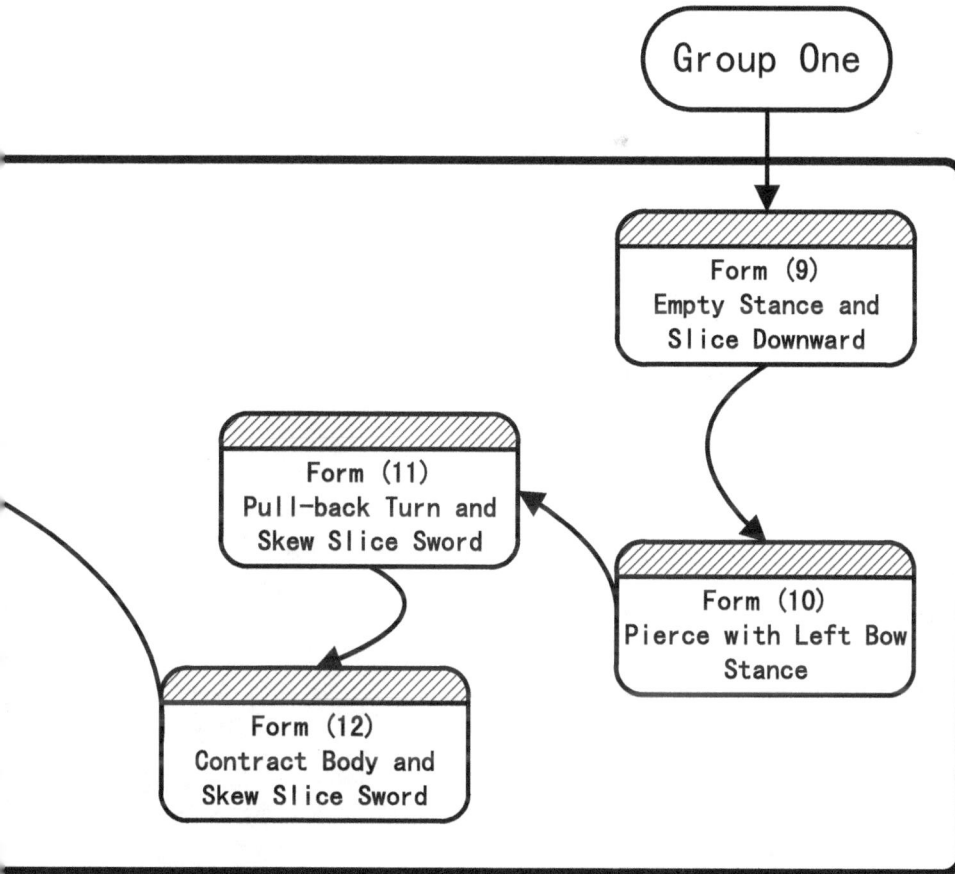

Group One

Form (9)
Empty Stance and
Slice Downward

Form (10)
Pierce with Left Bow
Stance

Form (11)
Pull-back Turn and
Skew Slice Sword

Form (12)
Contract Body and
Skew Slice Sword

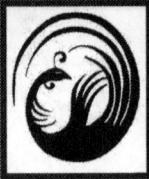

17. Form 17

In this form you change the direction to the southeast with your body rotation.

18. Form 18

You send out the sword to the east direction with a parallel step.

19. Form 19

After rotation, you face east with the left bow stance.

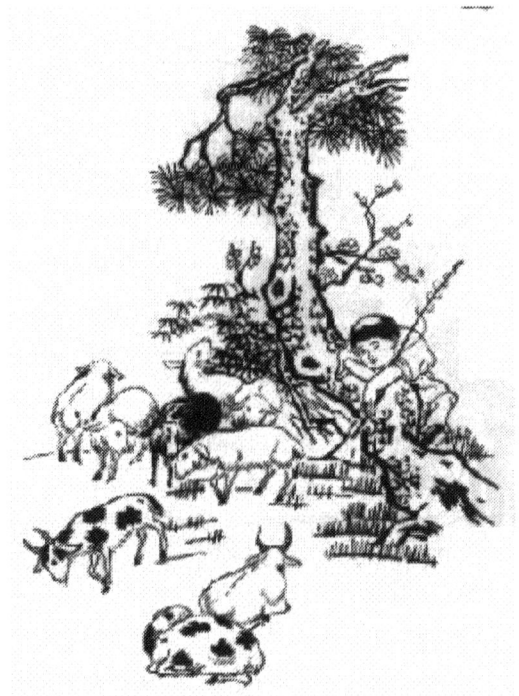

20. Form 20

After rotation, you face east with the right bow stance.

21. Form 21

After rotation, you face east with the left bow stance.

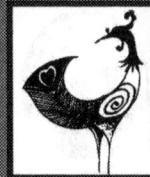

22. Form 22

Step forward and pierce your sword to the east.

23. Form 23

In this form, you change the direction to the west with the right bow stance.

24. Form 24

In this form, you sit on an empty stance and face south.

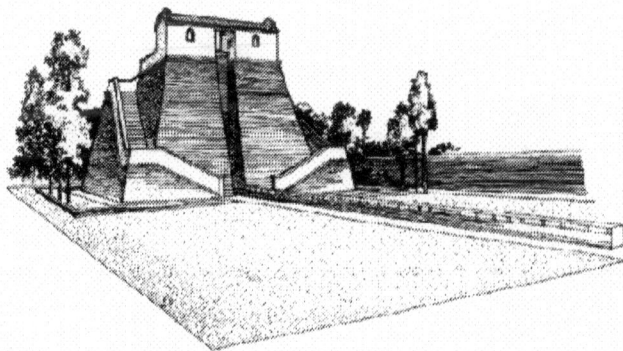

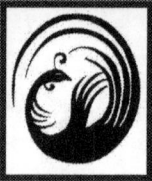

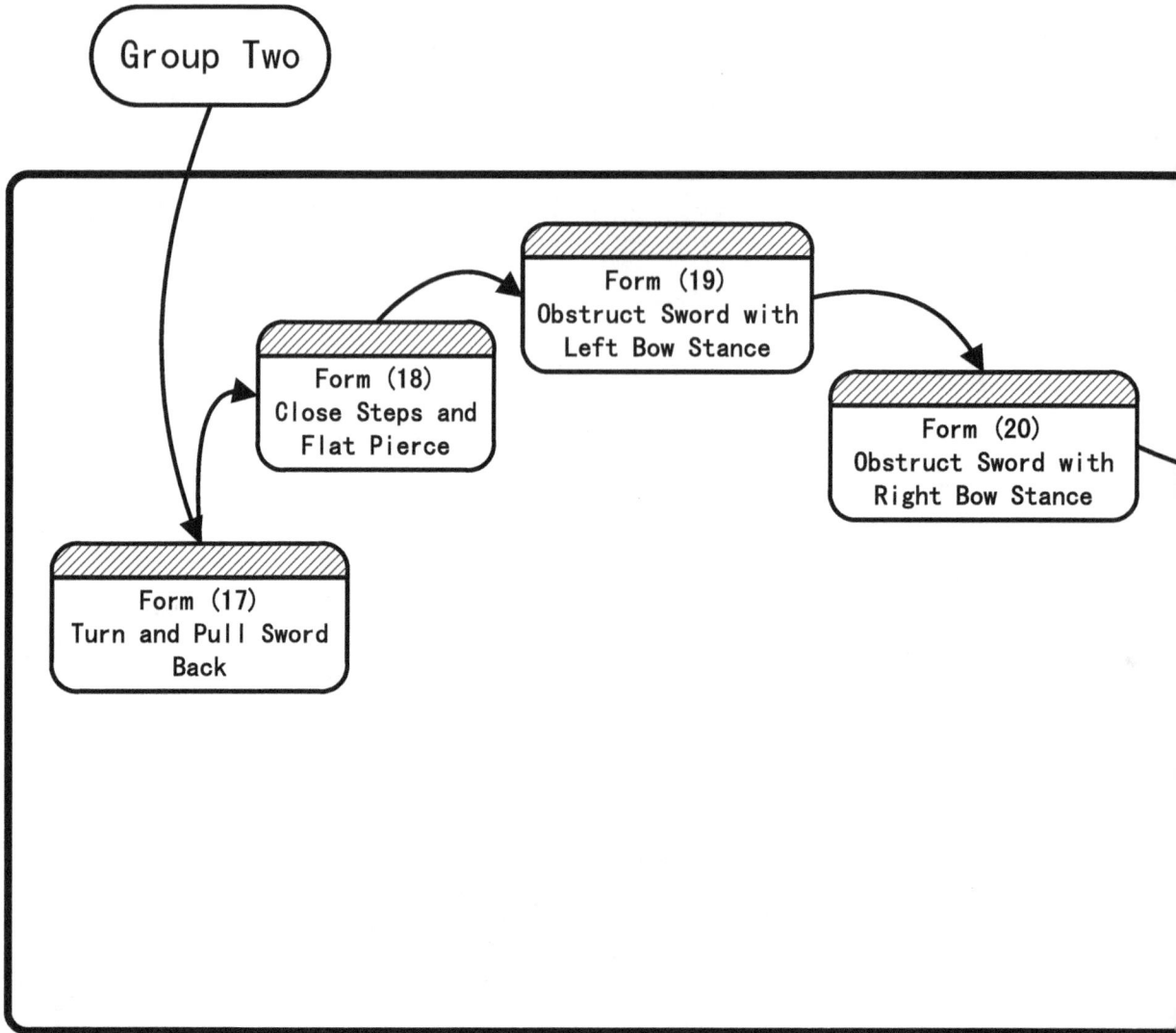

Group Two

Form (19)
Obstruct Sword with
Left Bow Stance

Form (18)
Close Steps and
Flat Pierce

Form (20)
Obstruct Sword with
Right Bow Stance

Form (17)
Turn and Pull Sword
Back

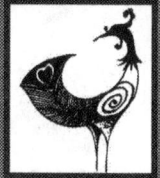

Group Three

Transitions

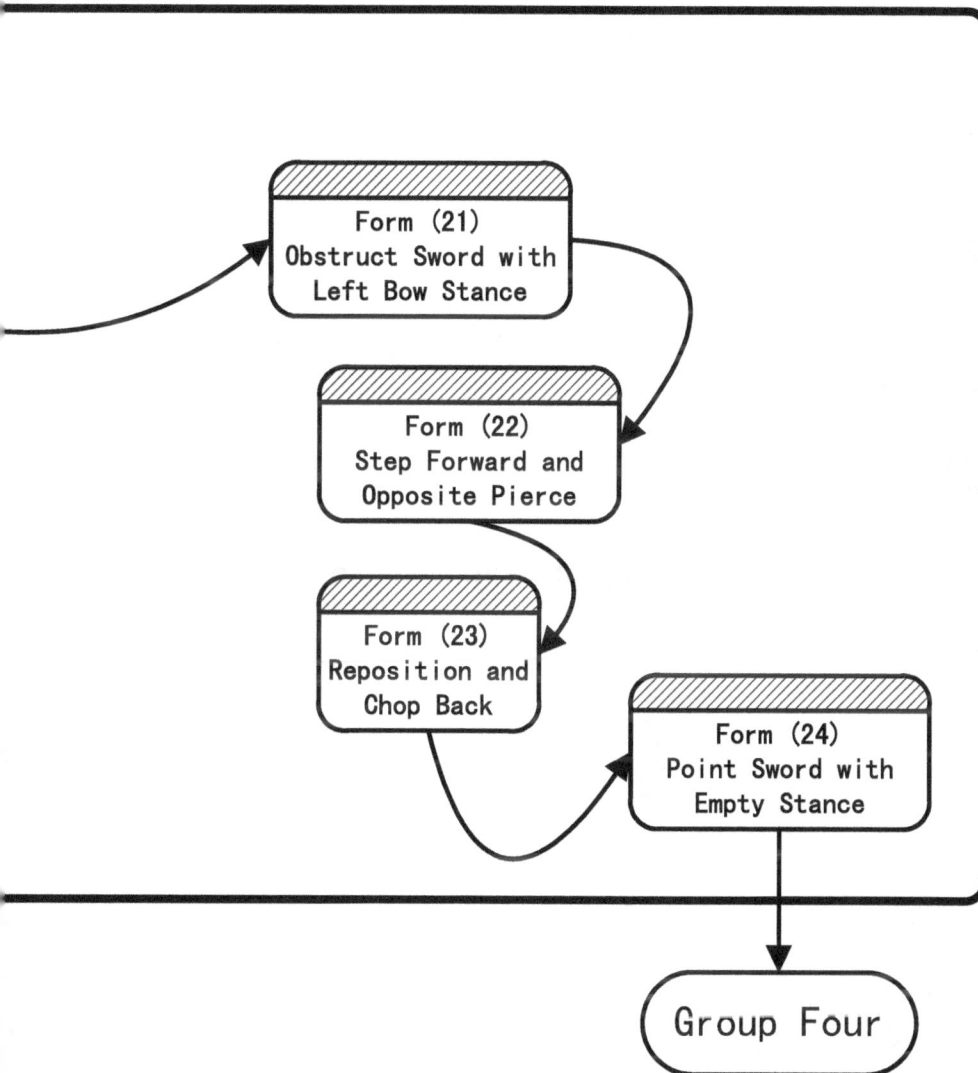

Form (21)
Obstruct Sword with
Left Bow Stance

Form (22)
Step Forward and
Opposite Pierce

Form (23)
Reposition and
Chop Back

Form (24)
Point Sword with
Empty Stance

Group Four

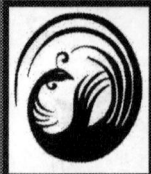

25. Form 25

In this form, hold the sword above your head with an independent stance to west.

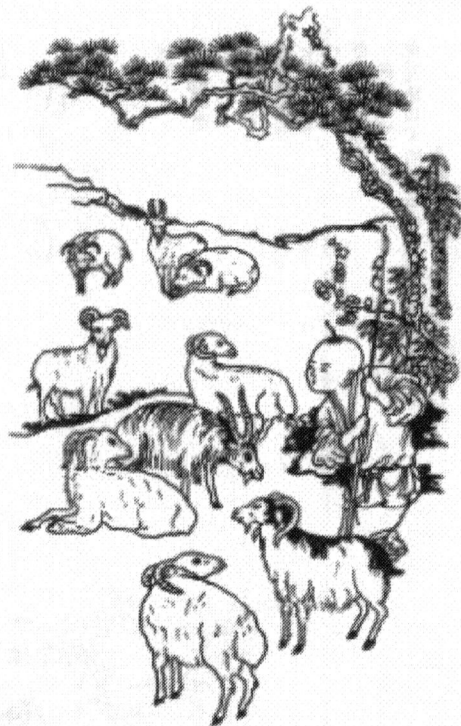

26. Form 26

Turn to the right bow stance and face west.

27. Form 27

Change to an empty stance and face west.

28. Form 28

In this form, you step back to face northeast.

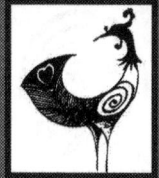

29. Form 29

After rotation, you send out the sword to the west.

30. Form 30

Change to the T-stance and face south.

31. Form 31

After 360 degree rotation, you face south.

32. Form 32

Pierce your sword to the south.

Closing Form

You pull both feet parallel and face south.

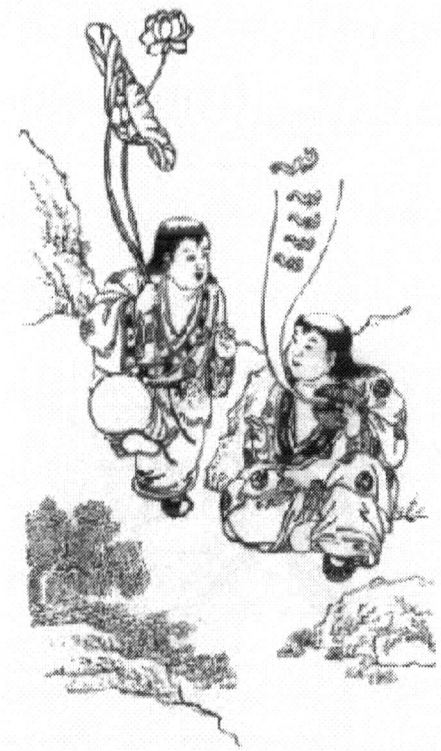

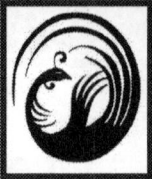

Group Four

Transitions

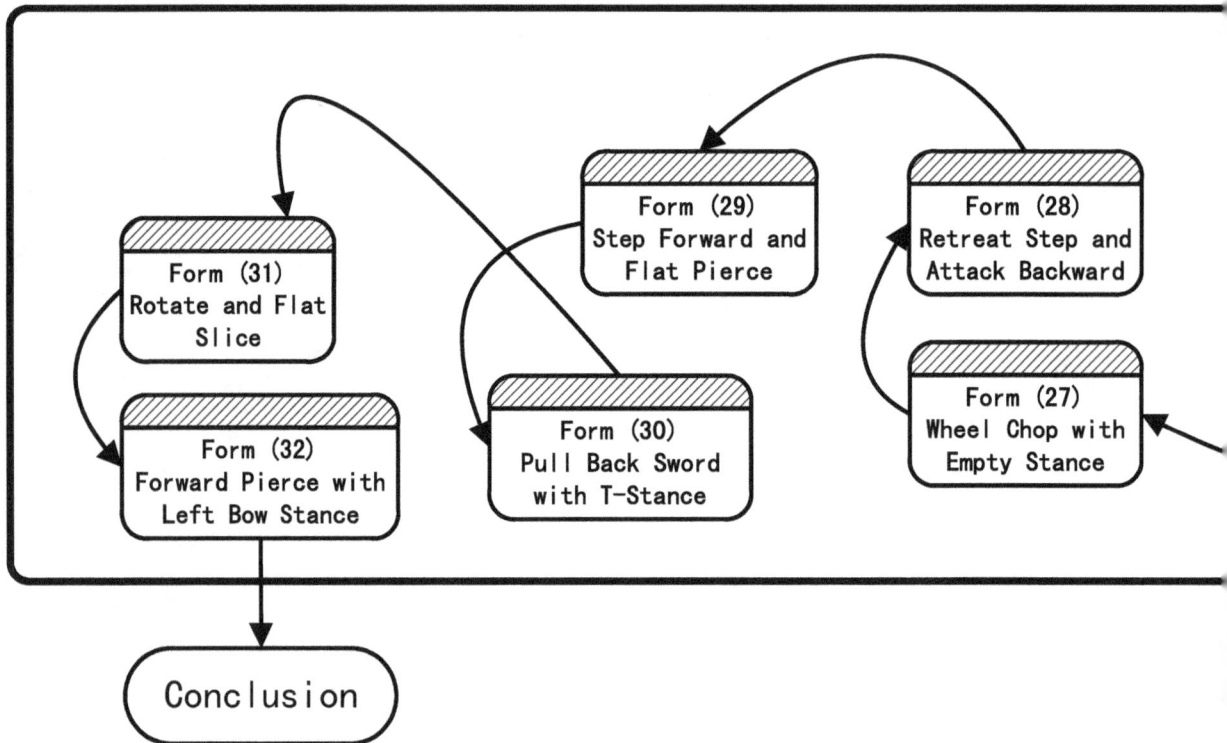

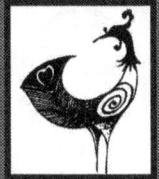

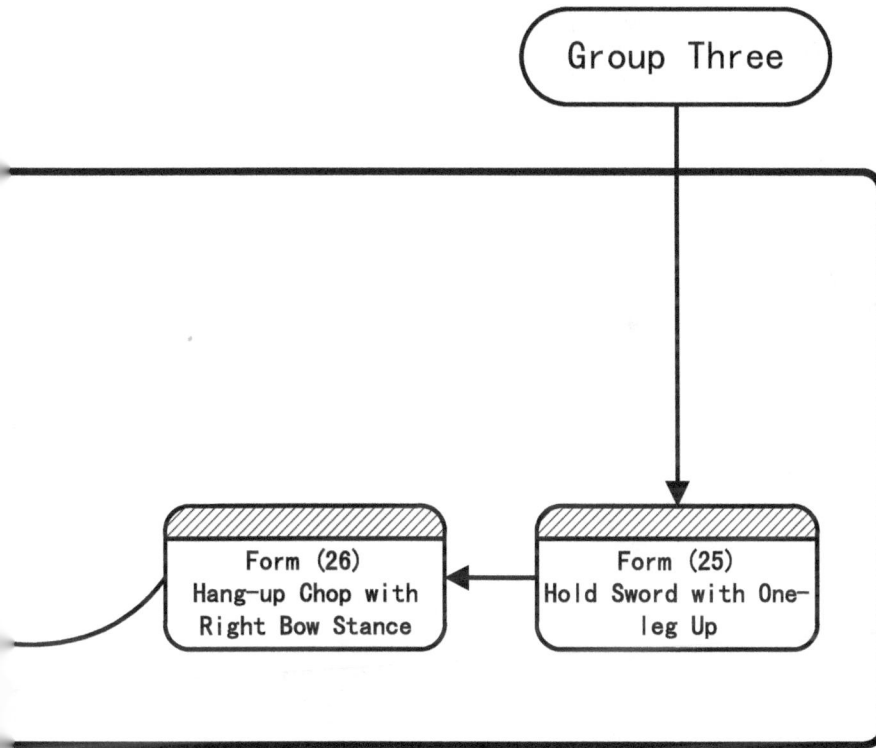

Group Three

Form (26)
Hang-up Chop with
Right Bow Stance

Form (25)
Hold Sword with One-
leg Up

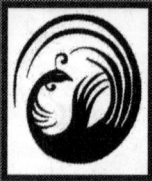

5

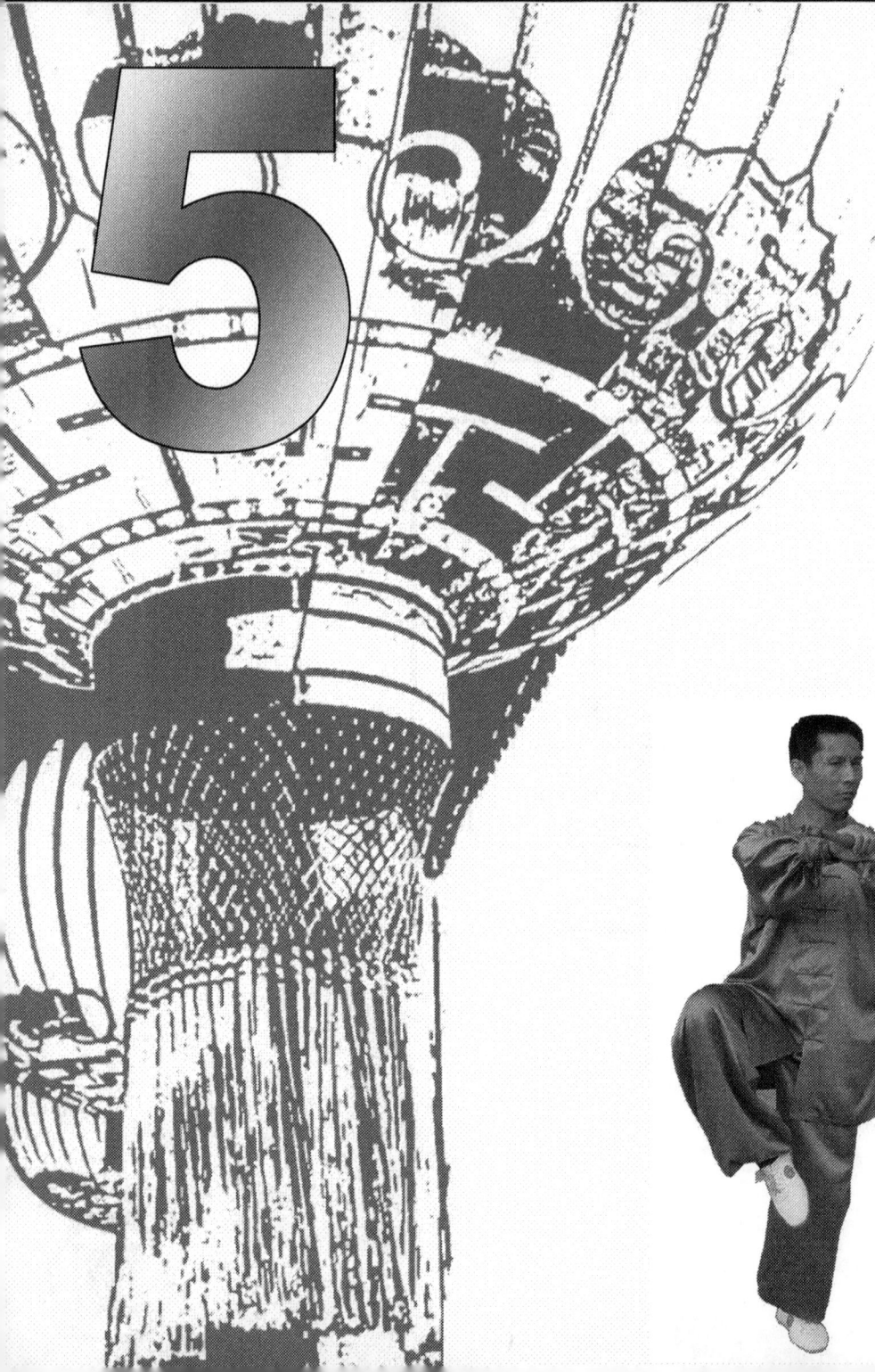

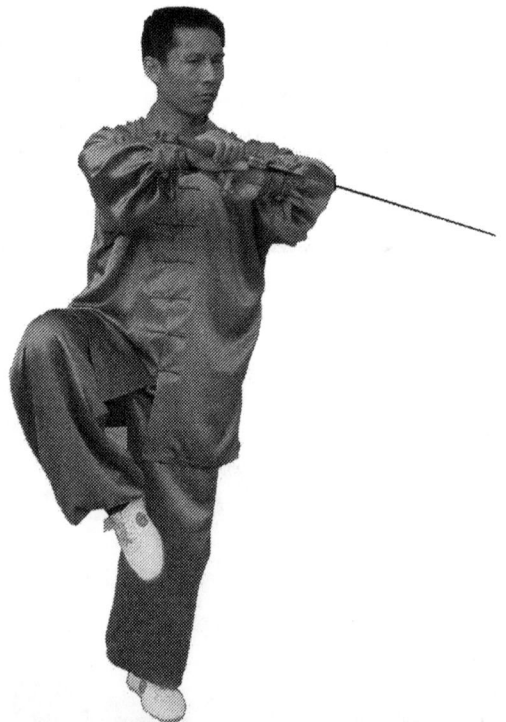

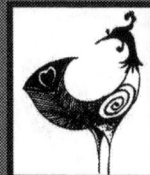

Chapter 5: The Fantasy in Tai Chi

Each of the 32 forms has a fancy name. This set of form names brings fantasy to Tai Chi Sword practitioners, in which the body and sword moves are somehow associated with the sky, sea, birds and dragons. For example, form No. 2 "Opposite Pierce with One-leg Stand" becomes "The Big Dipper Constellation"; and form 9 "Empty Stance and Slice Downward" becomes "Black Dragon Whips Its Tail". It is important to remember that Tai Chi has its deep roots in Taoism which has always taught people to learn from nature and become part of it. Many Taoists stay away from city and live a very simple life in remote mountains and villages. Nature is infinite and complex and powerful. This believe could be one of the reasons that many Tai Chi practitioners like to practice Tai Chi forms in the name of nature. Nature is so beautiful and does not need to change. We shall all come into accord. In the following, the fancy names of Tai Chi Sword are listed for those who practice in the spirit of Taoism.

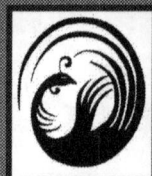

预备式 Preparation
起势（三环套月）Three Rings Circling the Moon

第一组（Group One）

1、并步点剑（蜻蜓点水）	Dragonfly Dips Water
2、独立反刺（大魁星式）	The Big Dipper Constellation
3、仆步横扫（燕子抄水）	Swallow Skims Over The Pond
4、向右平带（右拦扫）	Sweep To The Right
5、向左平带（左拦扫）	Sweep To The Left
6、独立抡劈（探海势）	Searching in the Sea
7、退步回抽（怀中抱月）	Embrace the Moon
8、独立上刺（宿鸟投林）	Sleepy Birds Returning To The Forest

第二组（Group Two）

9、虚步下截（乌龙摆尾）	Black Dragon Whips Its Tail
10、左弓步刺（表龙出水）	Green Dragon Emerges from the Water
11、转身剑带（风卷荷叶）	Wind Curls Up Lotus Leaves
12、缩身斜带（狮子摇头）	Lion Shakes Its Head
13、提膝捧剑（虎抱头）	Tiger Holds Its Head
14、跳步平刺（野马跳涧）	Wild Horse Jumps Over the Creek
15、左虚步撩（小魁星式）	The Little Dipper Constellation
16、右弓步撩（海底捞月）	Scoop the Sea Bottom for the Moon

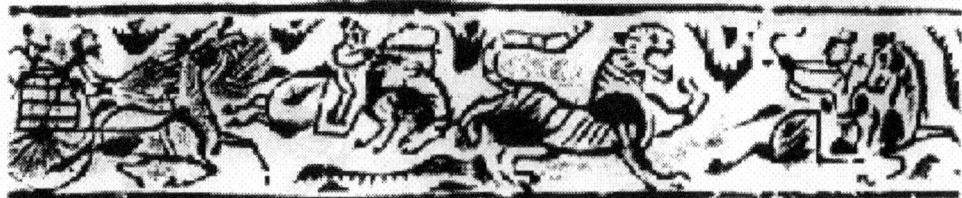

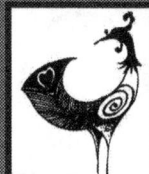

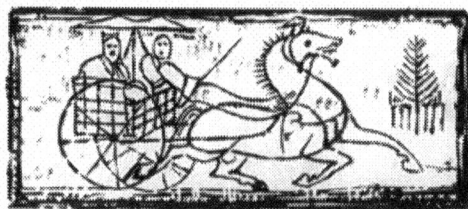

第三组 (Group Three)

17、转身回抽 (射雁式)	Shooting at Wild Geese
18、并步平刺 (白猿献果)	White Monkey Presents Fruit
19、左弓步拦 (迎风掸尘)	Dusting in the Wind
20、右弓步拦 (迎风掸尘)	Dusting in the Wind
21、左弓步拦 (迎风掸尘)	Dusting in the Wind
22、进步反刺 (顺水推舟)	Push Boat with the Current
23、反身回劈 (流星赶月)	Shooting Stars Chase the Moon
24、虚步点剑 (天马行空)	Heavenly Horse Galloping Across The Sky

第四组 (Group Four)

25、独立平托 (挑帘式)	Hook Up The Curtain
26、弓步挂劈 (左车轮剑)	Left Wheeling Sword
27、虚步抡劈 (右车轮剑)	Right Wheeling Sword
28、撤步反击 (大鹏展翅)	Phoenix Spreads Its Wings
29、进步平刺 (黄蜂入洞)	Wasp Enters Its Nest
30、丁步回抽 (怀中抱月)	Embrace the Moon
31、旋转平抹 (风扫梅花)	Wind Sweeps The Plum Blossoms
32、弓步直刺 (指南针)	Compass Needle Pointing South

收势 (Conclusion)

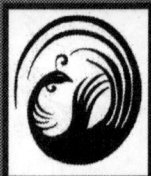

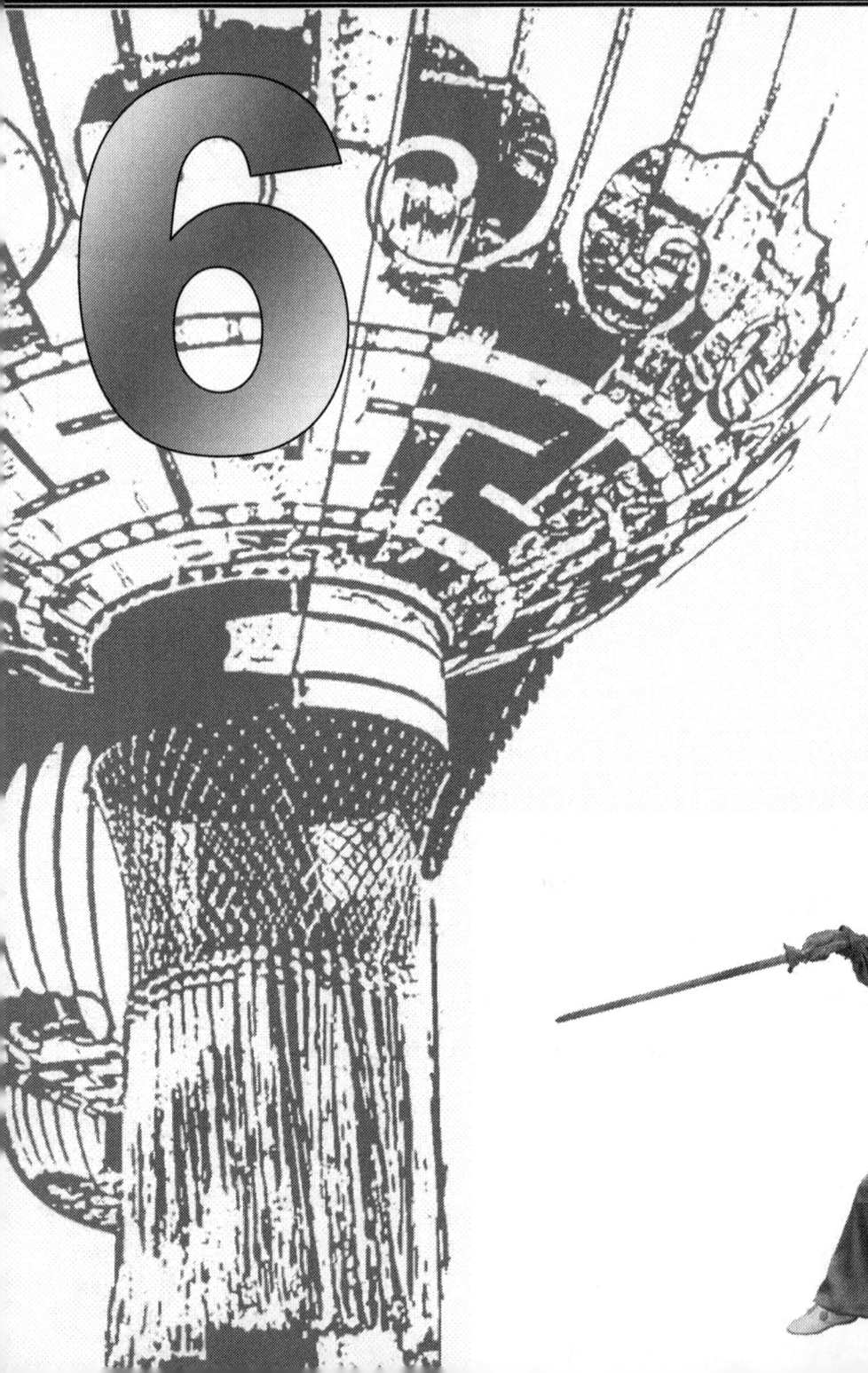

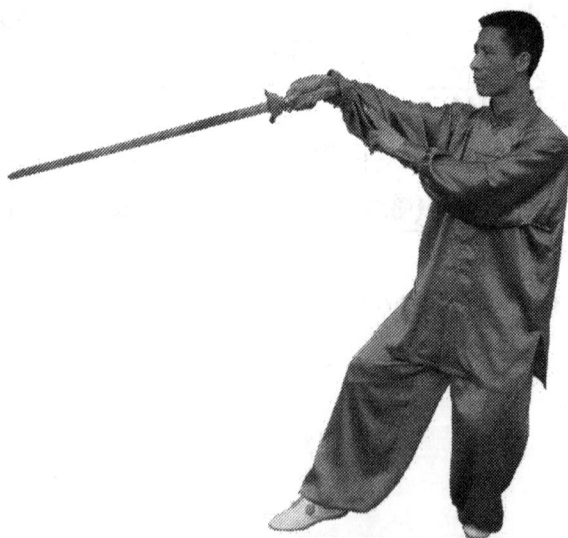

6

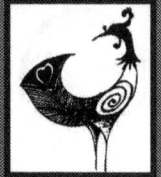

Chapter 6: Questions and Answers

In this chapter, several groups of questions will be answered. They are questions collected from Tai Chi classes, some of which were from beginners and somewhat were asked by students who have practiced a year or more and gained deeper understanding of the principles of Tai Chi. These questions and answers will help you see how others understand Tai Chi as an art of health exercise.

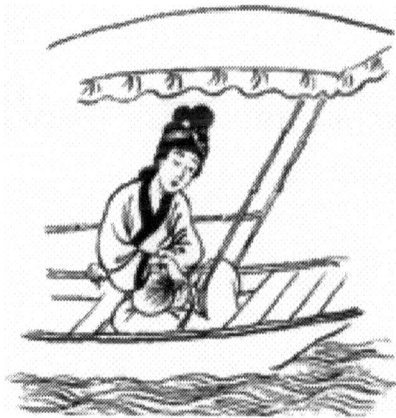

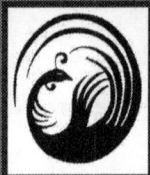
Questions

1. What kind of clothes and shoes should Tai Chi practitioners wear?

2. How much time should be spent practicing Tai Chi each day?

3. How to judge the quality of a person's Tai Chi Chuan?

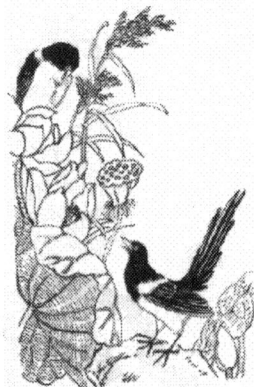

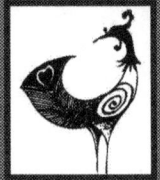

Answers

Q: What kind of clothes and shoes should tai chi practitioners wear?

A: Loosely fitting clothes and soft flat shoes, such as sneakers, will do.

Q: How much time should be spent practicing tai chi each day?

A: It depends. One must feel comfortable at the end of practice and not tired. One must not exercise too much.

Q: How to judge the quality of a person's Tai Chi Chuan?

A: To tell the quality of a person's tai chi form, just examine the following:

(1) The angles of the body when performing each posture and the transitions between each movement; (2) the pace of the movements; (3) the height of each posture. A person is considered a good practitioner when he/she can carry out every movement gracefully, with coordination and precision. A good tai chi practitioner keeps the same height during the execution of the forms. He/she does not bob up and down. The ending form finishes in the place the opening form began. The form is practiced in a constant and regular pace. The movements of the limbs should be coordinated with the waist. All postures should be erect, coordinated, continuous, flowing, and balanced throughout the forms. The whole body should be relaxed.

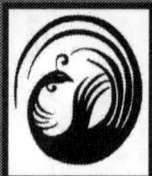
Question

What are the general principles in practicing Tai Chi Chuan?

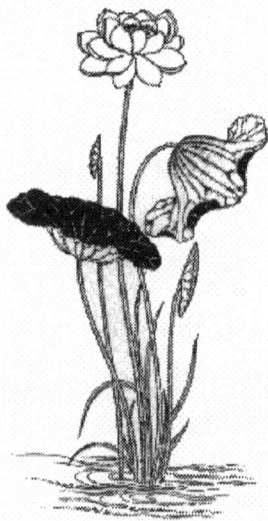

The following rules are attributed to master Yang Chengfu: Tai Chi Chuan 10 Important Points.

1. The spirit at the top of the head should be light and sensitive.

2. Sink the chest and raise the back.

3. Relax the waist.

4. Distinguish full and empty (substantial and insubstantial).

5. Sink the shoulders and drop the elbows.

6. Use mind not strength.

7. Coordination between the upper and lower body.

8. Internal and external unity.

9. Continuity without stopping.

10. Seeking stillness in movement.

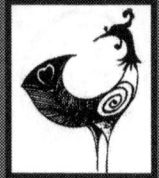

Answer

Q: What are the general principles in practicing Tai Chi Chuan?

A: In general, tai chi practitioner should follow the following rules:

1. The head energy insubstantially leads upward.

2. The eyes gaze with concentration.

3. Keep the chest in and raise back.

4. Sink the shoulders and drop the elbows lightly.

5. Keep body center straight, central, and upright.

6. Relax waist and thighs.

7. Both feet flat on the floor.

8. The top and bottom of the body are coordinated in a harmonized way.

9. Distinguish between fullness and emptiness.

10. Internal and external are harmonized with natural breathing.

11. Mind leads, not straight force.

12. All postures flow smoothly, the entire body is comfortable.

13. All postures should be centered and upright.

14. Keep stillness in motion and motion in stillness.

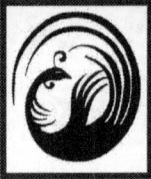

Questions

1. When people say: "The head energy in-substantially leads upward," what does it mean?

2. How do I understand the meaning of "The eyes gaze with concentration"?

3. Do I need to "Keep the chest in and raise the back lightly"?

4. Why do I have to "Lower and sink the shoulders and drop the elbows"?

5. Why do I need to "Keep body center straight, central, and upright"?

6. What am I exactly doing when they tell me to "Relax waist and thighs"?

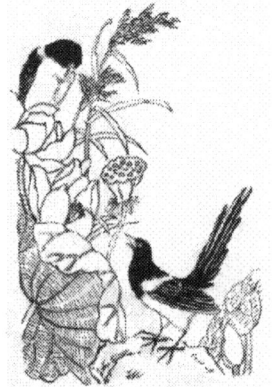

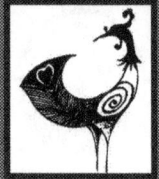

Answers

Q: When people say: "The head energy insubstantially leads upward," what does it mean?

A: The head feels like it is suspended from above. In this way, the whole body moves lightly and agilely.

Q: How do I understand "the eyes gaze with concentration"?

A: When a person's mind has concentrated, he/she will be aware even the slightest movement.

Q: Do I need to "Keep the chest in and raise the back lightly"?

A: The back has the feeling of being lifted lightly, and the chest is the slightly sunken. In this way, your chest is relaxed and the lungs move freely. So the answer is yes.

Q: Why do I have to "Lower and sink the shoulders and drop the el-
A: bows"?

Lowering the shoulders and dropping elbows helps with relaxation. This makes the transition easy.

Q: Why do I need to "Keep body center straight, central, and upright"?

A: The body's spine should be straight and erect, not leaning to the side.

Q: What am I exactly doing when they tell me to "Relax waist and
A: thighs"?

The waist commands all movements. Relaxation of your waist and thighs will make the connection between the waist and the knees easy.

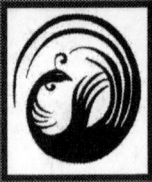

Questions

1. Why do I have to put "both feet flat on the floor"?

2. What is the meaning of "the top and bottom of the body are coordinated in a harmonized way"?

3. Why do I have to "distinguish fullness and emptiness"?

4. How do I understand the meaning of "mind leads, not straight force"?

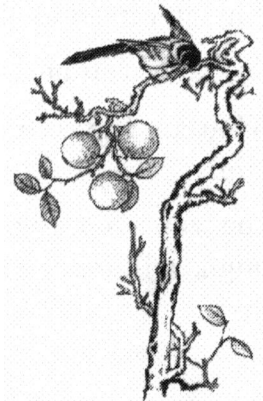

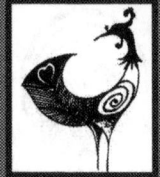

Answers

Q: Why do I have to put "both feet flat on the floor"?

A: The feet (or foot) must always be flat, sticky on the ground and relaxed, This is so that your body center will be rooted.

Q: What is the meaning of "the top and bottom of the body are coordinated in a harmonized way"?

A: The entire body must move in an integrated, coordinated way. Follow three harmonies: hands with feet; shoulders with limbs; elbows with knees.

Q: Why do I have to "distinguish fullness and emptiness"?

A: If one leg bears the major body weight, it is full; Otherwise, it is empty. It is critical to distinguish fullness and emptiness in order to gain agility.

Q: How do I understand the meaning of "mind leads, not straight force"?

A: This means you should think first before you move into the postures.

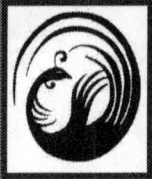

Questions

1. Why do some people tell me that "all postures flow smoothly, the entire body is comfortable"?

2. What is the meaning of "all postures should be centered and upright"?

3. It seems contradictory to "keep stillness in motion and motion in stillness", doesn't it?

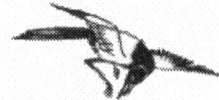

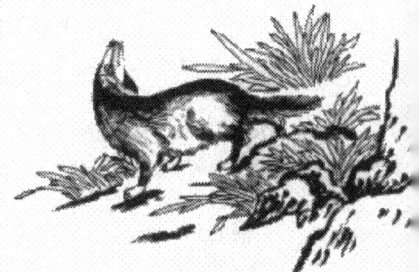

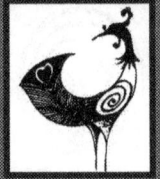

Answers

Q: Why do some people tell me that "all postures flow smoothly, the entire body is comfortable"?

A: All forms should be performed smoothly from the beginning to the end. There should be no breaks, jerks, or sharp angles. All movements should be natural and comfortable.

Q: What is the meaning of "all postures should be centered and upright"?

A: Your body should be upright, centered, balanced and coordinated. Your arms and legs should be neither too extended nor shrunken in.

Q: It seems contradictory to "keep stillness in motion and motion in stillness", doesn't it?

A: This means all movements are peaceful and flowing.

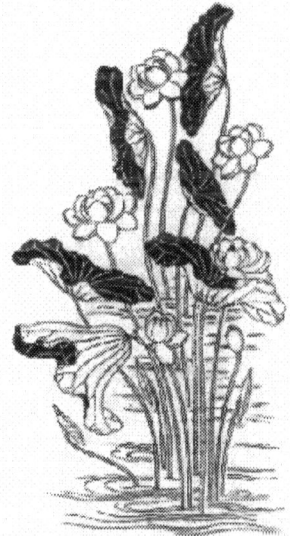

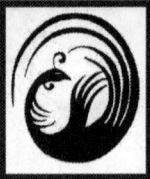

Question

How to breathe while practicing tai chi forms?

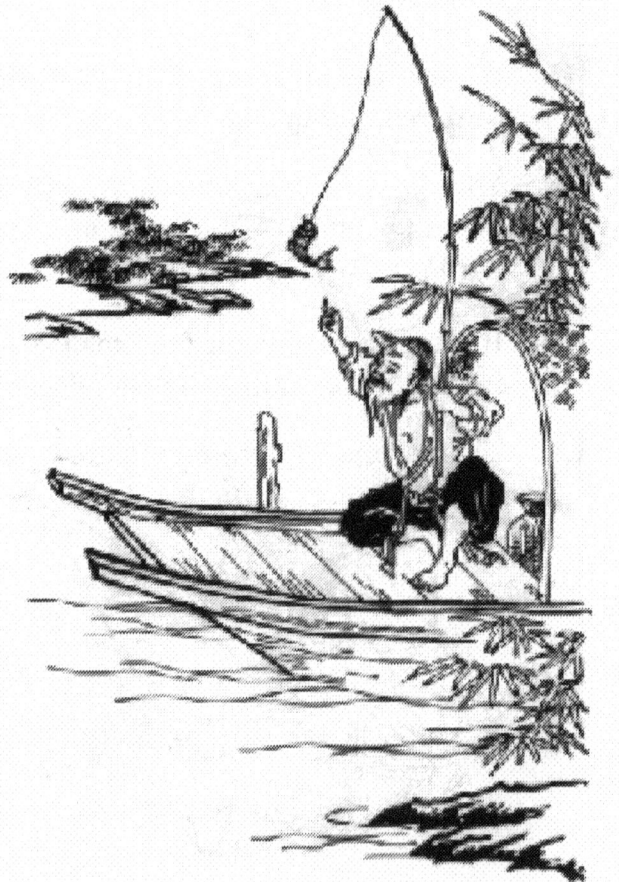

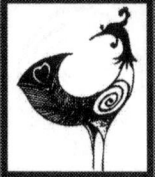

Answer

Q: How to breathe while practicing tai chi forms?

A: Breathe naturally. After training for a long time, one should be able to breathe according to the following rules with each posture:

1. open (inhale) and close (exhale);

2. up (inhale) and down (exhale);

3. raise (inhale) and sink (exhale);

4. back (inhale) and out (exhale);

5. squeeze (inhale) and extend (exhale);

6. shrink (inhale) and stretch (exhale).

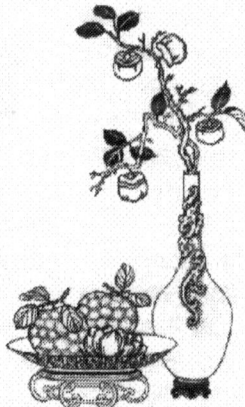

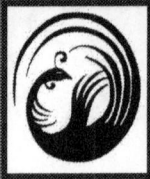

Reference

Feng Zhi Quang, The Encyclopedia of Tai Chi Chuan, Xuyuan Publishing House, Beijing, China, 2005

Tai Chi Chuan Sports, edited by People's Republic of China Physical Education Committee in 1996. ISBN: 7-5009-1150-5

Peter Lim, "Combat Yang Taijiquan", http://www.chebucto.ns.ca/ Philosophy/Taichi/ combat.html, June 14, 2006.

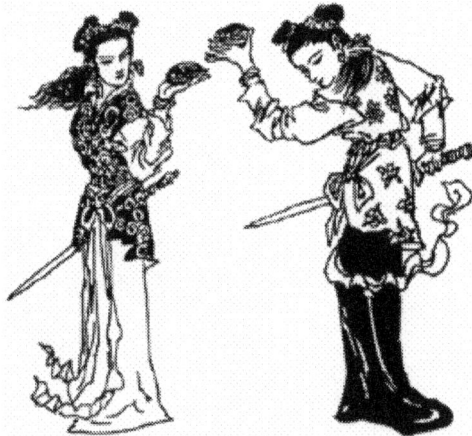

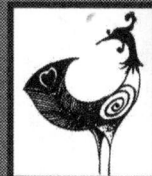

Index of Sword Forms

Monthly Workout

	Sun	Mon	Tue	Wed	Thu	Fri	Sat

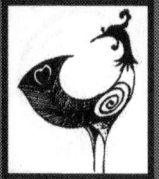

MONTHLY WORKOUT

Sun	Mon	Tue	Wed	Thu	Fri	Sat

Plan your workout

It is a good idea to plan your monthly workout schedule with your teacher at some point so that you do not miss any class. Use the calendar templates here to mark your schedule or photocopy them for your class.

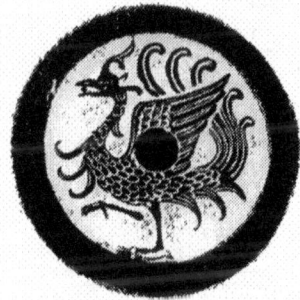

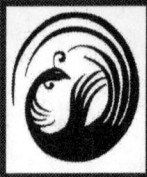
Tai Chi Accessory Order Form

Item #	Description	Qty.	Price	Subtotal

Order total: _____

Tax: _____

Shipping: _____

Total: _____

Name _____

Address _____

Phone _____

Method of Payment

☐ Check

☐ Bill Me

☐ Visa

☐ MasterCard

☐ American Express

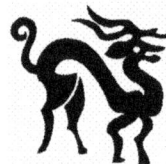

Credit Card # _____   Exp. date _____

Signature _____

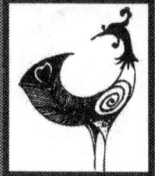

Name		Sign up for:		Time	Price
Address		☐			
		☐			
		☐			
		☐			
Phone		☐			
		☐			
		☐			

Method of Payment

☐ Bill Me   ☐ Visa

☐ Check   ☐ MasterCard

☐ American Express

Credit Card # _____ Exp. date _____

Signature _____

Subtotal: _____
Tax: _____
Total: _____

Special Offer

Teachers may use this book for Tai Chi classes. Tai Chi clothes or other teaching materials may be ordered from the TAI CHI instructors using the forms provided here. As a way of assisting Tai Chi teachers, two coupons are printed here for the promotional purpose of any Tai Chi classes.

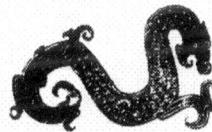

Write to Dr. Cheng Zhao about Tai Chi if you have any questions and comments.

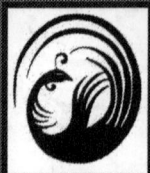

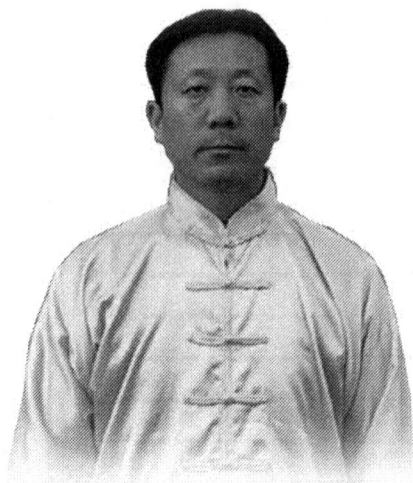

About Dr. Cheng Zhao

Dr. Cheng Zhao is a full professor at Indiana State University. He started his formal Tai Chi Chuan training more than 20 years ago in China. In 1987, he became a disciple of grandmaster Xin Yu He. Coincidently, Li Guang Qi and Dr. Zhao were in the same class on the same day. Cheng Zhao continues to learn and practice Yang style (Xin group) Tai Chi. To meet the interests of Tai Chi practitioners in Terre Haute area in Indiana, Dr. Zhao founded the Indiana Tai Chi Academy in 2005. He currently leads a group of Tai Chi practitioners to learn and practice Tai Chi Standard Forms; Tai Chi 24 Hand Forms; Tai Chi 32 Sword Forms; Basic Tai Chi Pushing Hand Forms; Traditional Yang Style (Xin Group) Long/Short Forms. He hopes through his teaching, many people will experience the art of Tai Chi and discover a genuine path for health and tranquility.

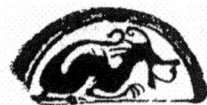

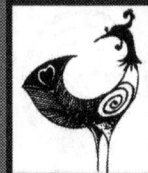

Write to Dr. Cheng Zhao about Tai Chi if
you have any questions and comments.

309 Woodbine Drive
Terre Haute, IN 47803
U.S.A.
Phone: 812-877-6328
E-mail: taichi.cheng@gmail.com

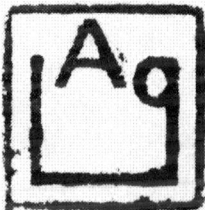

Agilceed Books
Knowledge changes life

Agilceed Books is a small publishing
company promoting the share and
exchange of the knowledge that posi-
tively affects people's life. Agilceed
Books firmly believes that the per-
sonal ownership of knowledge will be
more meaningful after the knowledge
has been expressed clearly and sys-
tematically in public and reaches the
people who need it. Agilceed Book
will continue to help people to publish
their knowledge in the right way.

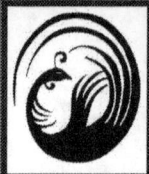

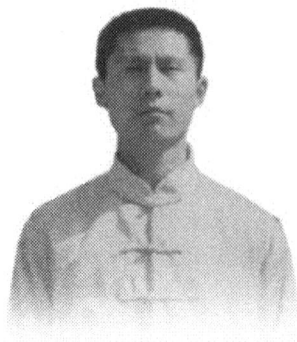

Li Guang Qi became a disciple of Grandmaster Xin Yu He in 1987. He followed Xin Yu He for 11 years and has taught and practiced Tai Chi in Jinan, Shandong of China for more than 20 years. He inherited and developed all grandmaster Xin style Tai Chi training. In this book, we would like to thank Master Li Guang Qi for allowing us to publish his Tai Chi pictures and his performance DVD for the first time.

Yang Style Tai Chi

Yang style Tai Chi was founded by Yang Lu Chan (1799-1872). His grandson, Yang Cheng Fu (1883-1936) is the third generation of the Yang family. He taught many Tai Chi students who later became famous. One of Yang Cheng Fu's leading disciple was Li Ya Xuan (1894 - 1976). Li's famous disciple was Liu Zhong Qiao whose last disciple was Xin Yu He. Master Xin spent 9 years learning Tai Chi from Liu Zhong Qiao and reached a very high level in Yang style Tai Chi at the end of class. He founded his Yang style (Xin group) Tai Chi in Jinan, Shandong Province of China. The current leader of Xin group Tai Chi is Master Li Guang Qi.

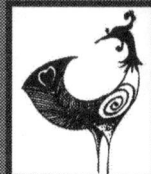

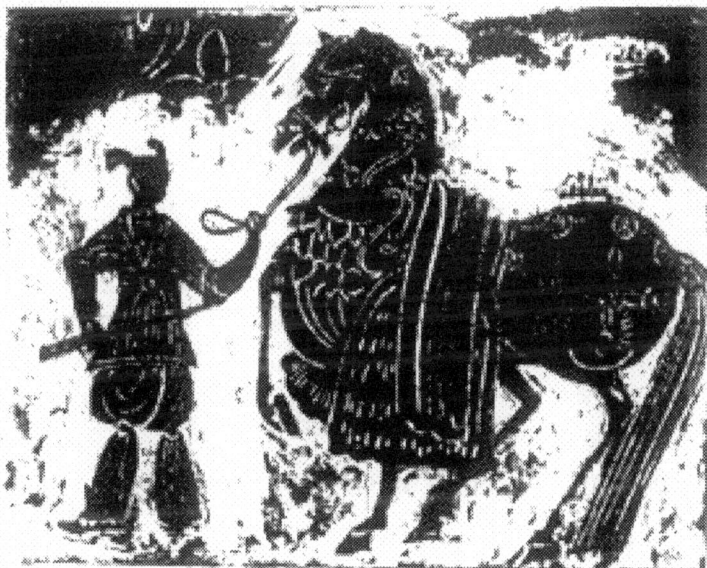

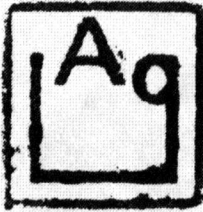

ISBN	ISBN-10: 0-9761183-2-7
	ISBN-13: 978-0-9761183-2-9
SIZE	7.5" x 9.25"
EDITION	1st. Ed.
MANF	TSWD-327
PUB DATE	2006-10-16
TRACK NO.	V1-6A160